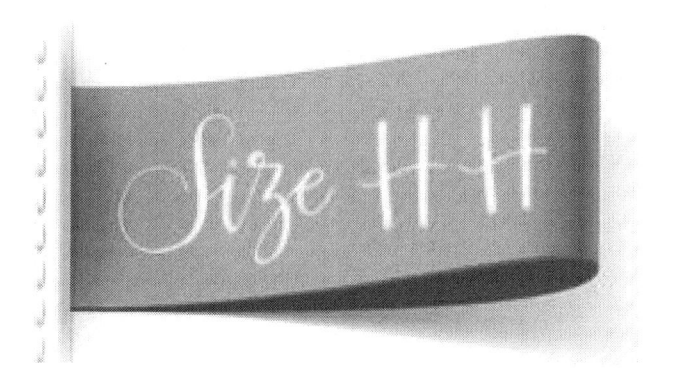

The most enviable size to be…

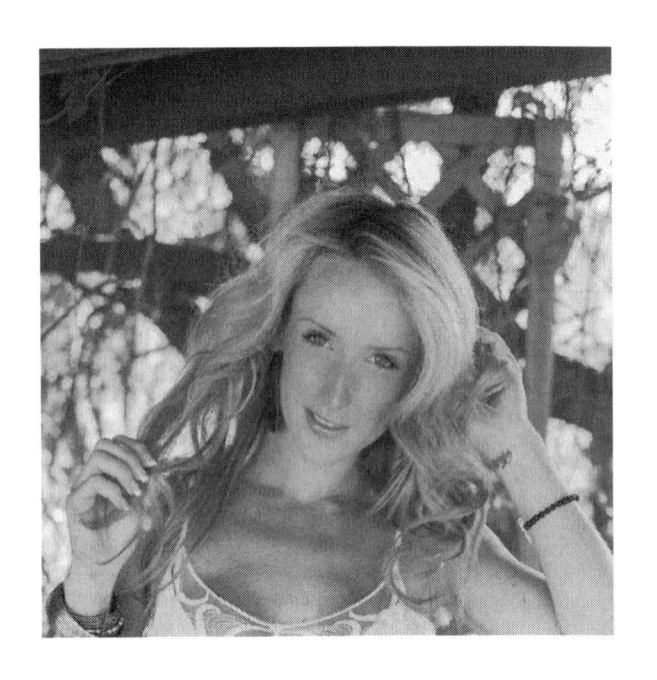

By Eva George

Published by Eva George
Copyright 2015 © Size HH
Editor ~ Jacqui Malpass
Cover design and Illustrations ~ Mercedes Lopez Charro
Contributors ~ Alison Francis, Natalie Guyan, Caroline Ferguson, Jane Travis, Jacqui Malpass
Author photo ~ Agata Jensen

This book is not intended as a substitute for the medical advice of physicians. The reader should regularly consult a physician in matters relating to her health and particularly with respect to any symptoms that may require diagnosis or medical attention.

ISBN: 978-0-9935000-4-6

Dedicated to my two daughters. May happiness, health and confidence fill your hearts every day. Unconditional love from mum x

Contents

The Mind ~ Where the changes start	1
Lifestyle ~ Small Changes Lead To Big Results	27
Nutrition ~ A good body is made in the kitchen	55
Exercise ~ Stretching, Posture & Toning	109
Overall Points To Remember	137
Acknowledgements	141

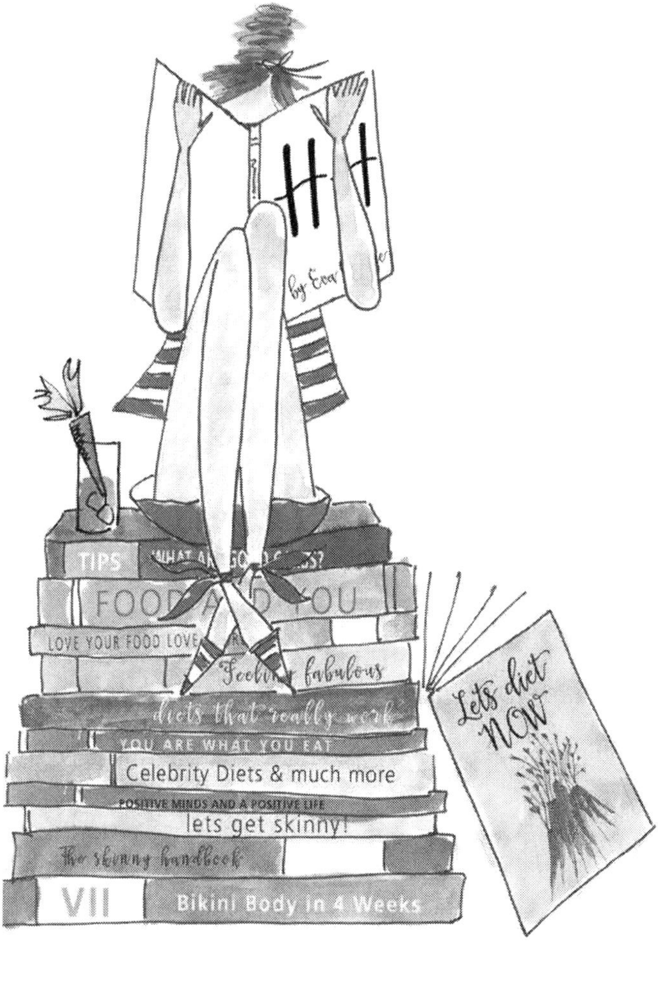
TIPS
diets that really work
YOU ARE WHAT YOU EAT
Celebrity Diets & much more
POSITIVE MINDS AND A POSITIVE LIFE
lets get skinny!
the skinny handbook
VII
Bikini Body in 4 Weeks
Lets diet NOW

Welcome to size HH. Grab a cuppa and make yourself comfy.

You will find this book helpful if you are a serial dieter and tired of the struggle, or you feel a failure for not being able to stick to diet plans.

Many of us are too busy to find the right way to eat or don't have time to eat as well as we would like. You might even be someone who thinks they cannot afford to eat healthily or someone whose lifestyle means pounds have been piled on, and can't see a way to change.

You will also find this useful even if you have reached your desired weight but would like to tone up, or even just to feel more confident with yourself and figure.

WHAT IS SIZE HH?

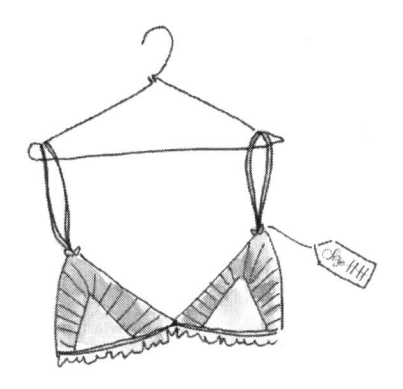

It sounds like a generous bra size doesn't it? Size HH simply means to be **Size Happy and Healthy**. Imagine the hilarity of telling your friends that you are working towards size HH - **happy and healthy.** I bet they will want some of that too…

My name is Eva George, and I discovered size HH after having my first child. Before pregnancy, I was never particularly happy with my body and was always finding fault. It was a habit that I had since the beginning of my teenage years (like many of us).

As a child, I had always led a very active lifestyle, winning school sporting events and running at local races. However, just before I reached my teens, my body, lifestyle and emotions started to change. I eventually dropped out of sports and started smoking, drinking, partying and eating whatever I wanted; takeaways, kebabs, you name it, I ate it. The total opposite of what I had been taught and needed as a growing girl! It wasn't long before I started to hate the way my body (and mind) was changing from lean and strong to soft and weak.

Little did I know my body shape was *supposed* to be going through huge changes at that age, *regardless* of my eating and exercise habits. I didn't know it was perfectly normal to put on body fat in some areas, in preparation for hips and bust, during the whole 'growing up phase', so I did everything I could to fight it.

Cutting a long story short, reaching adulthood, the feelings I *still* had for my body drove me to quick-fixes, diets, extreme exercise, and I was on the brink of developing an eating disorder. I became very thin, even landing some modelling work, but despite the media's portrayal of thin as beautiful, I still hated myself and felt unhealthy.

The extreme dieting led to bad skin, dry hair, frequent mood swings and low mental and physical energy. After completing some basic nutrition, anatomy and physiology courses in college, things changed... a little.

I learnt the right things to do to keep healthy, but like many with great knowledge I didn't always follow the advice. My mind was not in the right place, and my lifestyle was hectic with different jobs, traveling, studying and a social life. I was living mainly on ready meals, noodles, cereal, toast and chocolate, even though I knew how bad it all was for me. It was quick and easy though!

After settling down and falling pregnant, I finally began looking after myself for my baby's sake and fell in love with my growing bump. I started to aim for healthy rather than skinny which was a *huge* change in my habitual thinking. I was determined to be happy and healthy for my baby. I realised I could stop finding fault with my figure now, as long as it is healthy then what else really matters!? Carrying something precious was my wake-up call and the discovery of perspective. It was like the last piece of the puzzle for me. For others and for you, it may be a totally different reason that will lead you to becoming Size Happy and Healthy.

I discovered it takes a simple combination of factors to achieve a healthier body and mind **quickly**, so I want nothing more than to share what I have learnt, because it works! Losing weight is not our main goal because it doesn't guarantee health or happiness. You could lose all the weight you wanted on the scales, but if your mind still isn't in the right place, you will feel no different. Health is our main goal because it's the foundation for all happiness! Weightloss (or weight gain in some circumstances) just happens to be a side effect of becoming Size Happy and Healthy, if our lifestyles have led us to becoming too overweight, or underweight for our natural balance.

We are swamped with ads for the latest diet fads, pills, and workout DVDs. While they all have their place, **they do not work long term**. Our internet feeds and magazines are filled with beautiful models of a certain size, the latest diet and weight loss trends, and stories about who weighs what, or who lost their baby weight quickest - making us think that *this* is what's important.

The beauty of being human is that we all come in different shapes and sizes. We are meant to be unique! One thing we could all have in common though is size HH. Being able to squeeze into a size 0 dress does not necessarily mean happy or healthy, believe me, so let's forget traditional clothing sizes. This book is about loving the unique shape and person that you are and bringing your body and mind to its full potential!

Everyone knows a well-balanced diet and regular exercise are the **healthiest** ways to lose excess body fat. This is often easier said than done though because more often than not, the mind, habits, beliefs and/or lifestyle gets in the way!

I meet many people who want a quick fix, the same as I did, but the trouble is quick fixes rarely last. Some of these extreme diet methods mess up your metabolism so badly that you end up putting more weight back on afterwards, so the cycle, known as yo-yo dieting continues.

If you are a yo-yo dieter, you need to know - and believe - that long-term weight loss, happiness and great health is possible. To get out of the cycle, you need to:

- Adopt a **sensible plan with plenty to eat,** so you know you can stick to it
- Know your strengths and weaknesses
- Most importantly, be willing to change your mindset

The rest of this book will show you how to start making positive changes to your mind-set, body and lifestyle, today.

Image counts for a lot in this world unfortunately, but it's not everything; health is far more important!

By committing to reading this book and following the advice, you have already taken the most important steps towards a happier and healthier new you, and that's what counts.

Size HH is a place to start and a place to turn when you want to make new healthier changes in your life. It's about finding and maintaining the **right weight for you**, accepting the *shape* you are and learning to love living in your body, for the rest of your life.

We are going to focus on the four key points you need to shape up physically and mentally and be as healthy as you can be (without spending a fortune or hours at the gym). After all, we only live in these bodies once, why not treat it like a princess and feel as good as possible? Your body will thank you in later life, guaranteed! Don't think you are too old to start to do this either!

Only read on if you have made the decision that you are prepared to start feeling differently about yourself in a healthy and happy way, today.

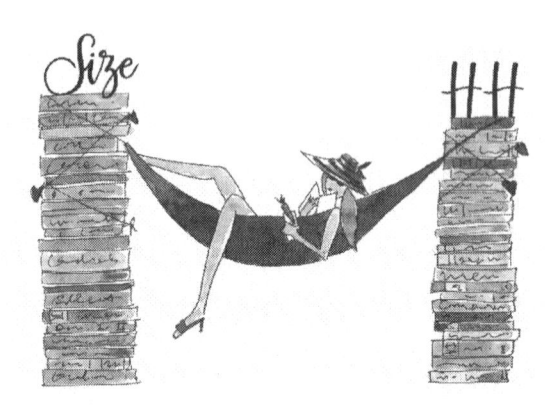

If you are not ready, just keep me safe and pick me up when you are looking for a change…

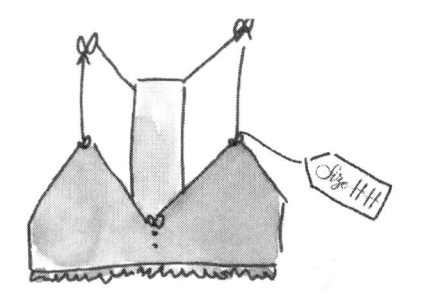

THE MIND – WHERE THE CHANGES START

Eva George

~ Natalie Guyan's Story ~

Natalie's story is typical in many ways, apart from one. Unlike most serial dieters, she eventually found the right way to lose the body fat that was causing her issues, keep it off and become size HH for life.

"Back then, I had no choice. I'd always struggled with being "big boned" and what with my thyroid being underactive, I thought I'd never be able to lose the weight I'd rapidly gained while pregnant. Besides, I *had to* eat more because I was breastfeeding (so I thought). You see, it had absolutely nothing to do with the hearty meals I was making every night. It really didn't matter that my portion sizes were huge, or that I'd wash my dinner down with a few glasses of wine and maybe a cheeky ice cream, crisps or chocolate bar after. I found traditional workouts boring and was sure it wouldn't work for me anyway, what with my big bones etc. When trying on clothes, I was totally convinced that the shops were now making sizes smaller. I wasn't a size 22!! I'd always been a 14...

My younger sister on the other hand, (I was sure) was genetically blessed. She enjoyed going to the

Size HH

gym! When she told me that maybe I was eating the wrong foods, or too much food and asked if I was happy, she was just trying to get into an argument, wasn't she?! That nurse at the hospital when I had chest pains suggesting I should lose some weight was just being bitchy, so I thought!

But then I saw a photo of me taken in New York right after my husband proposed. It wasn't me in the picture, it couldn't be. It didn't look like the normal size 14 me. I didn't want to be the person in the picture. I certainly didn't want to be a plus size bride! It was my wake-up call and a chance for me to accept some guidance.

My sister suggested to start by keeping a food diary so I could make myself aware of what I was actually eating… what an eye opener! Turns out I was polishing off between 3-4000 calories a day, significantly more than the additional 500 recommended when breastfeeding. I was now fully aware that what I was eating was directly affecting the way I looked, my health and my mental wellbeing. The food didn't just miraculously disappear once I'd eaten it…. Everything has an after effect and the evidence was staring me in the face.

I was given a book for Christmas later that year. It had all my favourite recipes in it but with ways to make them healthier. There was a website too, with lots of other ladies just like me. No judging, just a group of gals who loved food and wanted to make a change. The website recommend I dropped my calorie intake to just 1400 per day, so I switched to low cal, low fat foods as advised. The inevitable happened and my weight loss plateaued. Overnight I'd dropped my calorie intake by half. Of course I lost some weight on the scales, but I was tired, grumpy and constantly hungry. The recommendation was to go even lower cal but I there was no way I could stick to it and so my weight crept back up. The solution? Weight loss patches and diet pills! Sure I was full of energy buzzing off the occasional shakes from all the caffeine (and who knows what else in them). I even lost a few pounds, but they found me again quickly when I stopped the pills and patches.

After trying various diets and experimenting with every product and weight loss solution I could put my

Size HH

hands on, I lost a few more pounds. They didn't stay gone though and the scales kept drawing me back for more judgement. I just couldn't keep it up and it was affecting all areas of my life.

Seeing me at breaking point, my sister persuaded me to go for a run with her. I ran 50 yards! I walked the rest. Later on though when my heart rate returned to normal and I stopped sweating like a pig, I genuinely felt better for it (even slightly proud of myself). Feeling all revved up and motivated, it even inspired me to join a gym.

The motivation didn't last long though. I was a slow starter and didn't enjoy the gym at all. Eventually, I got bored and decided to try out a few different exercise classes instead. The weight was coming off gradually, but I wanted faster results now I was on a mission to slim down. Everyone was recommending running!! Euergh!! I hated running, but I knew I had to try it, so I signed up for a 1/2 Marathon to give me something to aim for and hit the treadmill to begin training. When I started, I could only run for 30 seconds at a time before feeling out of breath, but eventually that became 18 minutes, 30 minutes and then one hour! Signing up for the race had given me a strong reason not to give up. I completed the half marathon I set out to do in 2hrs 28mins! I then went on to complete a 10k race in 54minutes, a very respectable time and something I never thought possible!

A few months later, I found out I was pregnant again; I was over the moon, but fear set in that I was going to gain all my weight back, by this point I was five stone down! Despite my best efforts, I regained some weight, around two stone in total. In a bid to lose the weight as quickly as possible, I went on a popular high protein, low-fat diet. It was gruelling, but I lost the two stone, plus one more, in just three months. However, I was then left with lots of excess skin and a serious case of the grumps! I had reached my goal weight but I was still far from being happy or healthy. All the extreme dieting, running and endless hours of cardio had taken its toll. I was starting to resemble a deflated balloon, eating less and less, and afraid of carbs. Even fruit was a rarity! My health was hanging off a cliff all in the name of wanting to lose weight!

Size HH

I thought I knew everything there was to know about dieting and food, but after meeting a personal trainer friend and being completely honest with them about my struggles, I realised I was missing the vital link. I didn't need to be depriving myself and living on the bare minimum anymore; I needed to eat to fuel and nourish my body with foods that would give me energy, a better state of mind, make me strong, protect me from illness and keep me active. I needed to find the ultimate balance, not starve myself to lose weight.

I've learnt a lot along the way; how to prepare my favourite meals in a more nutritious way and being active and exercising should be fun!

By trying lots of different sports and activities I've found what works for me, I've met lots of great new friends and above all, I know that whatever I do, it's because I'm in control of the choices I make. I'm responsible for me. I choose to be happy and healthy.

Aiming for strong and healthy rather than skinny works for me. The stronger I feel, the more motivation I have to keep going and do better, improving myself even more. I have gone beyond levels I thought I could, and my body has surprised me!

Food wise, I currently eat around 2,500 healthy calories spread over 5-6 meals a day because it suits my lifestyle. Nuts, seeds, avocado, coconut oil and olive oil are all staples. Around 50% of my diet is made up of healthy fats, the other 50% is a mixture of fruits, rice, oats, sweet potatoes, free range and grass fed meats, fish and of course the occasional cake or biscuit if I fancy it! This works for me. Now to find what works for you!

Exercise wise, these days (When I am not challenging myself to lifting a heavy deadlift bar) I still don't find running very enjoyable and instead prefer brisk walking with my sister, daughters and husband, taking in the local scenery, adventuring up hills and catching up on the gossip. I find a walk genuinely stimulating and even stress relieving at times! It also keeps my cardio fitness in check and is a great fat burning method, without being too harsh on my joints."

The good news is that like Natalie, you can change and relearn how to look after yourself, in the

Size HH

very best way. Regardless of the reason you put on weight in the first place, there is one thing that everyone's body responds well to. That is good nutrition and a positive mindset.

BECOME AWARE OF YOUR THOUGHTS

The mind is undoubtedly one of the most important tools for shaping up and becoming happy and healthy. When your **thoughts** and focus are in the right place, motivation and willpower comes easily. Not only that, but your thoughts become actions. Actions become habits and habits become your life. The great news is; **you control your thoughts**, not the other way around. Are you keeping yourself from Size HH with your thoughts?

LOOK IN THE MIRROR AND LEARN TO LOVE WHO YOU SEE

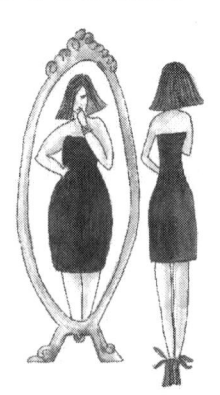

Size HH

We have all had days where we look in the mirror and don't like what we see (or conveniently dodge mirrors all together!). When we feel confident in the way we look, it makes us feel happier in ourselves, and we radiate more positivity towards others. So take a minute to look in the mirror and appreciate the things you DO like about yourself; eyes, hair, teeth, bust, whatever it is.

Every day when you look in the mirror, only focus on what you *like* about your body and style. Before you know it, you will have more and more things you like about your reflection and the way you feel in your clothes.

TRY THIS

A great exercise would be to stand in front of the mirror wearing something you feel good in, (or at least very comfortable in) and make a mental note of at least three things you like about your reflection.

Do this for at least seven days and you will notice the positive effect. It's amazing how once you start to notice your best bits, that's all you will see because suddenly the attention is taken away from your 'not-so-good' bits. The negative feelings you had will be become weaker as the good feelings become stronger; that's why it's important to acknowledge things you like about yourself as well, even when you are not in the mood.

COMPLIMENTS

We tend to be very modest when we receive personal compliments about ourselves, with a huge percentage of us not always believing the compliment anyway. It's helpful to accept any compliment graciously, even if you don't fully believe what they say. Replying with thank you and returning a compliment is an instant bonding between two people and a rush of positive energy for you. If someone were to say something negative about you, would you take it straight to heart and keep going over it in your mind? Probably. So do the same with a compliment.

SOCIAL DECORUM

As women, we are known for bonding and even creating friendships over the dislike and criticism we have for our bodies. It's always nice to have someone in the same boat who understands what we are feeling! Sharing the struggle of not being able to lose weight, or sympathising over stretch marks and mum tums. It can be comforting to know we are not alone. We are usually great at finding things we like/love about other people, but it has become almost socially unacceptable to like/love things about ourselves (or at least admitting to it) without appearing 'full of yourself'.

When we encourage body positivity and loving yourself, we don't mean going around telling everyone you are the best thing since sliced bread. We mean just finding and acknowledging your plus points too because there is nothing wrong with that! What makes you unique? Find, acknowledge and appreciate things you like about you so you can bond and create friendships by helping each other feel better, then they can aim for being healthier with you!

THE WHEN I MIND GAME

Another mind game we play with ourselves is pondering over the 'When I' statement… Are you guilty of thinking to yourself "I will be happy **when I** am a size …."(You fill in the blank). If so, you are convincing yourself that you won't feel good until you reach a certain size or weight. And with those thoughts you won't, because the mind is very clever! *Remember, your thoughts become reality*! **You are still 'you'** whatever your size or weight. Break this pattern of negative self -talk by thinking of all the reasons you have to be happy and just concentrate on those!

Most people think the transformation is what leads to being happy and of course it does, but being genuinely happy *first* is actually half the transformation already.

If you change your focus from 'losing weight' and only aim to be as healthy as possible, the **right size for your shape** will come as a result!

Good feelings bring motivation and energy! Imagine you are wearing a fabulous new outfit, or have just had your hair done how you like; it instantly makes you feel more alive! This powerful, positive feeling is what we want more of. That's why it's important to make the decision to start feeling as good as you can about yourself… **right now** - whatever shape, size or weight you happen to be at the moment.

Size HH

Of course, this is easier said than done for many of us. Yet it can be as simple as consciously replacing negative thoughts with good ones as quickly as possible, before bad thoughts turn into bad emotions.

For example; If you think to yourself:

'I feel like a ten-tonne whale in these jeans.'

'I need to lose weight; then I will be happy.'

'If only my stomach were flatter.'

'I wish I could lose weight, but I love my food.'

These thoughts will obviously make you feel awful. So, as soon as they come into your head, replace them with something that makes you feel more positive such as:

'I am lucky to be alive to see the day.'

'I have a loving personality that this worlds need more of'

'My brain is my superpower and it will help me get through anything!'

'The strength of my body and mind is unknown, even to me, so they should never be underestimated. Especially by me!'

Forget those naughty negative thoughts as quickly as they come in. They do not serve any purpose. Even start humming a song you love, or the theme tune to your favourite TV show as soon as the old habitual thoughts pop into your head. Anything other than thinking about things that will wreck your mood! When you feel dispirited, that is a signal from your emotions to your brain to say:

"Attention brain! Please think something happy, you are spoiling the party!

TRY THIS

Many find it useful to use journaling to express and become more aware of what they are thinking and feeling, even helping to manage conditions such as depression and OCD. It only takes a few seconds, but the results can be very interesting and quite emotionally relieving.

> *A journal is a written record of your thoughts, feelings, experiences, and observations. You can write in your journal daily, or only when you feel the urge. Journaling is the act of keeping, writing, reflecting and making personal change through the art of keeping a journal.*

Size HH

If you think this might help you, invest in a pretty journal and see where your mind takes you!

For any of you reading this who may be suffering from depression (diagnosed or not), we understand that being happy is not always as easy as just thinking positive, or eating and sleeping better, it's just not as simple as that (although all these things help to manage it). Depression is a medical condition caused by an imbalance of chemicals in the brain (mostly serotonin), with sufferers of all ages. It is more than just feeling upset or down. Just because Size HH is a positive book, does not mean we will sweep this issue under the carpet, it's more common than many of us care to admit.

The great news is, depression may not be permanent, and your doctor can help you find the right treatment for you to help you recover and figure out what your triggers are. It is very important to have treatment for depression as soon as possible so that it doesn't lead to chronic mental illness.

Eva George

STAY POSITIVE AND SWERVE THE SCALES

The scales can be misleading. In fact, the scales tell awful fibs! Still many of us cannot resist going back to them for judgement on a regular basis. The problem is, after all of the dieting, we are usually disappointed with what they say. Women's weight constantly fluctuates. Remember that women retain several pounds of water prior to menstruation. This is very common, and the weight will likely disappear as quickly as it arrives. Which means it's pretty impossible to get an accurate reading if you weigh yourself too often.

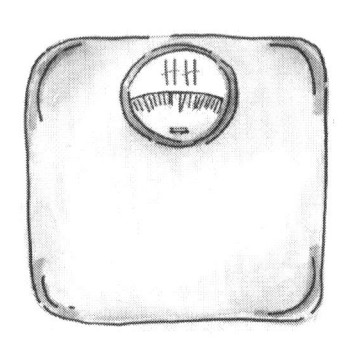

Size HH

When you constantly look at the scales, hoping to see that all important number, your mind becomes influenced in a negative way if you don't see the results you want. This could lead to even more dieting and leave you nutritionally deficient, unhealthy and unhappy. So, to stay as positive as possible from now on, ditch the scales, unless you own a set that specifically measure body fat, water, muscle, etc. In which case only weigh yourself once per month and keep in mind, even the expensive scales are not 100% accurate. The best way to track your progress is with a good old fashioned tape measure! It is more tailored to your individual shape and will help you stop trying to force your entire body down to a certain weight or size.

BE YOUR OWN CHEERLEADER!

If you have made the decision from this point forward to be happy and size 'healthy', then that is what you will be. Think of it as your mantra and repeat it often. You don't need to tell anyone you are on a diet because you are not. You are just becoming the best version of you. Your friends, family and work colleagues, will be amazed by the positive results! Have faith in yourself!! Never let your negative thoughts create a vicious cycle of bad emotions in your life. Otherwise, things, unfortunately, will not change. From today after reading this book, you WILL feel better about your shape/size/body/weight. Even if you find this hard to believe right now!

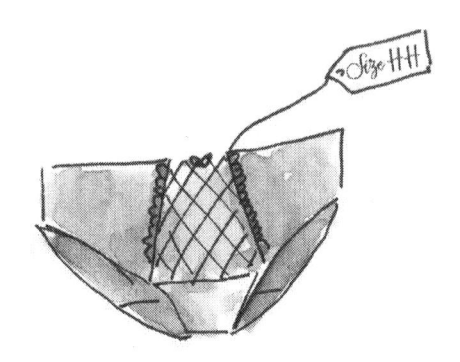

Size HH
FIND YOUR MOTIVATION

The next step is to find your motivation for becoming Size HH. Is it a wedding or holiday you want to shape up for? Maybe you want to be as slim as you once were, for health reasons, or you would like to set a good example to your kids, etc. Whatever it is, take a picture of it, or write it down and place it somewhere you look every day (the fridge is usually a good place!).

What other things leave you feeling motivated? What other things genuinely make you happy and smile? Start thinking about these... Even writing them down, or creating a vision board with photos and positive quotes may help.

For those of you that want a challenge, look out for the 30-day HH challenge online, where among other things I show you how to make an online vision board to kick-start and maintain your motivation.

Quote from Caroline Ferguson, Mindset Trainer.

"One reason why people lose weight and then regain it is because their motivation style is taking them in the wrong direction.

If your motivation is to MOVE AWAY FROM your uncomfortable state (e.g. I don't want to be fat or feel unattractive any more), this can work quite well to spur you to take action in the first place. But, as soon as you make a little bit of progress (e.g. losing 10lbs) and no longer feel the acute pain, shame and discomfort, your motivation drops, boredom sets in and you end up sliding back. Motivation to move away from a current state or situation is known as 'Stick Motivation'.

You can achieve much more sustainable momentum if your motivation is about MOVING YOU TOWARDS (rather than move away from) a strong and tempting vision of how great you'll feel and look when you reach your target health and fitness levels. This gleaming vision of genuine happiness and health is called 'Carrot Motivation' and it's a much more effective way to motivate yourself for the long haul. If you combine your mouth-watering vision with a clearly defined goal, an action plan and the right support, you can really fly."

Size HH

So, is your motivation about Stick (not wanting to be fat any more) or Carrot (wanting to be leaner, happy and healthy)?

YOUR BODY IS AMAZING

Of course, it's not always as simple as thinking positive thoughts. When you indulge in certain things that you enjoy and make you laugh, endorphins and dopamine, (the brain's feel-good chemicals) are released into your blood stream making you feel great. This also happens when you eat foods you enjoy. (I knew there would be a scientific reason for me craving those choccy digestives!) I can guarantee you though, the natural highs from being size HH are far greater than the short-lived highs of eating junk food.

Whenever you have a moment of weakness and think about giving into an old habit, **focus on your motivation**! Besides, there are healthy foods (and exercises) that release the same uplifting feelings too!

FOOD IS NOT YOUR ENEMY

There could be an underlying reason why you seem to be craving certain things like sugary foods. We will look into that more in the nutrition section.

Food doesn't have to become your enemy; you can still have things you enjoy – life is too short not too. Just remember *everything in moderation*. What you eat affects your state of mind in so many ways.

Good food = a better state of mind.

DON'T HATE, APPRECIATE

After reading this book, don't look back. Only forwards towards the healthiest version of you. The only time you should look back is to see how far you have come.

Just for a moment, think of all the hours spent disliking yourself in your head. Now imagine what it could have been like if you had been putting all that time and that energy into ways to feel good instead! You can't turn back the clock, but you can certainly use your energy in a better way going forward, and I will show you how in the rest of the book.

THE MIND POINTS TO REMEMBER

- Positive thoughts bring motivation and good emotions. Fact. So think more of them!

Size HH

- When you feel bad about yourself, distract your mind with something that makes you genuinely feel good; pets, children, music, photos, memories, or anything else that helps you to feel more upbeat.
- Traditional scales can be disheartening and put you straight onto a downer if you don't see the results you want. If you like to weigh yourself, only use scales that measure your body composition (fat, muscle, water levels, etc) for a more accurate reading of your progress. **The best way to measure your results is with a tape measure.**
- Have faith in yourself that you WILL be happy and size-healthy now, even if previous attempts haven't worked.
- Find your motivation for becoming Size HH and place a reminder of it somewhere you look every day.
- Carrot motivation means moving towards your vision (rather than moving away from a current state) this will help you maintain your efforts long term.
- If you regularly feel the need to snack on junk food, remember this. Eating addictive, highly

processed foods might make you feel good at the time, as they taste amazing, but they basically they have no benefits for your body whatsoever, only negative side affects. The high you experience is very short lived and in the long run you will feel even worse, absolutely guaranteed!

- If you want to enjoy sweet foods, you must have a well-balanced diet to compensate for them. Better still, swap unhealthy treats things for healthier versions, one by one. Train your taste buds to like better-for-you options. No one is asking you to cut them out of your life altogether! However, the healthier food you eat, the quicker you will become size HH and stay that way.
- You have come this far to read this book. You are ready to start the change. Now. Not tomorrow, not next Tuesday, no excuses. Now.

Now we have the mind in the right place, let's get started on the rest...

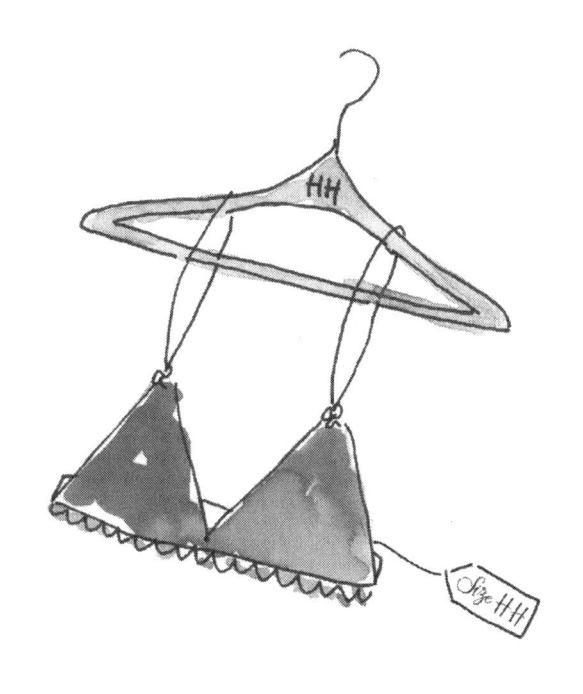

LIFESTYLE – SMALL CHANGES LEAD TO BIG RESULTS

Eva George

A friend of mine, when in her 20's, left home to live with her partner. She didn't know how to cook properly and resorted to ready meals, takeaways and comfort cheesy pasta dishes, all served up with bottles of wine. Combined with cosy evenings on the sofa and little exercise, it led her to become a little more 'soft round the edges than usual'. As she started to notice her favourite jeans tightening up, she became more obsessed with her weight and began dieting secretly to try and obtain the taught, toned figure that she had been used to.

During this time, the ladies she worked with fretted over her weight as they saw her arms and face becoming thinner, so they would buy her Belgian buns and other treats (She didn't have a sweet tooth, but ate them to keep her work friends happy and her dieting secret). Getting ever more concerned with her weight, she confessed to me that her lunch for about a year was a banana and a hazelnut yoghurt. And she started to exercise obsessively.

Later she was diagnosed with irritable bowel syndrome She says *"At no time did I attribute this to my dieting, lifestyle or stress. My cooking had improved, I was extremely fit (training 6-7 times per week) and ate in a way I considered to be healthy. However, by now I was constantly looking for the next miracle 'drug', which would improve my energy levels and keep me slim. Popping whichever supplements and weird potions I heard would work."*

After her relationship ended, her weight rose to ten stone, which she considered to be FAT for her figure!

Now, with only herself to please, she lived on toast with lashings of butter, jacket potatoes and processed, convenience foods. In desperation, she joined her first slimming club and religiously counted calories until she reached the magical nine stone mark on the scales. Being on her own she started to party and guess what? She didn't put on weight, but became very unhealthy and unhappy! Her lifestyle had gone to pot. She was convinced she was unattractive and refused to look in the mirror.

This is another example that reaching your dream weight on the scales may not keep you happy for long and that being a lower weight does *not* necessarily mean you will be any healthier.

LET'S GET SOME PERSPECTIVE

Before we go any further, I would like you to take a photo of yourself from the front, both sides and from the back. If you want to go more into detail, you could also take measurements of your waist, hips and each thigh to measure your progress as we go on. You don't have to show anyone, but without the photos and measurements, our brains may not notice the changes.

Remember to try and stay off the scales if you have a habit of using them regularly.

HOW DOES YOUR LIFESTYLE AFFECT YOU?

What positive changes could you start making today?

You don't need miracle diets, or pills that promise to make you slim. You just need to make new habits in your lifestyle. The time to start is right now.

BECOME AWARE OF YOUR HABITS

I found the best way to change my habits is to become more aware of the unhealthy habits I had formed and make a decision to change each of them, one at a time. If you took just one habit, made some alterations to your behaviour, interrupted the pattern and did that regularly for a few weeks, you would, I guarantee, see your habits change. Then take another habit and implement small changes around that for several weeks and so on. **Small steps work**.

TRY THIS CHANGING HABITS EXERCISE

Take a look at one of your habits and see if any could be made healthier. For example, you may find that when you're feeling lethargic you instantly reach for chocolate. A choccy bar or similar sweet snack will give you a quick sugar rush and feels like it really hits the nail on the head for about 15 minutes. Then the energy rush subsides and in a short space of time, you will hit rock bottom again! If you're feeling lethargic, it's a good idea to quickly scan through your body while asking these questions;

- What thoughts am I having?
- What emotions am I feeling?
- Am I actually thirsty or hungry for 'proper' food?
- Do I *really* need this chocolate bar, or am I just giving in to habit?

You may think nothing else in your fridge or cupboards will have the same satisfaction as your favourite chocolate, biscuits or cakes, but you may be pleasantly surprised to learn otherwise! I am a self-confessed chocoholic, and no amount of reading health books will change the fact I enjoy it. To save my body from the effects of regular love affairs with this man-made luxury, I have found other, healthier ways to curb and satisfy my choccy cravings, which I will share with you in the nutrition section.

Mindset Trainer, Caroline Ferguson, offers some valuable tips on how habits are formed and how to change them.

"During your lifetime, you develop thousands of habitual ways of thinking, feeling and behaving. Habits – good and bad – are continually being formed, strengthened and weakened. But why does it happen, and how?

You brain contains 100 billion nerve cells (neurons) which make connections with thousands of other cells. Whenever you do, think, or feel anything, electro-chemical impulses zip down a chain of interconnected neurons at up to 120 metres per second (nearly 270 miles per hour!).

When a nerve impulse travels down the same chain of neurons several times – as happens when you repeatedly think a particular thought or behave in a particular way – those neurons cement themselves together and form a 'road', which allows the repeated thought or action to happen more easily and become automatic. Those roads are known as neural pathways. Another word for a neural pathway is a **habit**.

Repetition isn't the only dynamic at play in the creation of habits. When you mix repeated thoughts and actions with *emotions*, habits develop more quickly and more deeply. Whether the emotion is positive or negative, the presence of feelings like happiness, joy, anxiety and guilt sends a signal to your unconscious mind: *"This is important, pay attention."*

This emotion factor is the reason why comfort eating can exert such a strong grip. When you eat a food that's high in fat and sugar (such as sweets or biscuits), your body releases feel-good chemicals that are as powerful as heroin. If this happens when you're feeling unhappy or stressed, the high can temporarily lift you out of that dark place.

Your unconscious mind files away this information and the next time you feel down, it sends a message to your body in the form of a craving for sugary food to lift your spirits. So you have a repeated behaviour paired with powerful feelings, which results in an emotional eating habit being formed.

The problem is that after the high comes the crash, as your body is flooded with insulin to metabolise the excess sugar. You plunge straight back down again – even lower, in fact, because now you're throwing negative feelings like guilt and shame into the mix, due to feeling bad about your loss of control.

Why, you ask, would your mind deliberately create a habit that's not good for you?

Unfortunately, the part of your mind that governs comfort eating isn't rational and doesn't make the connection between eating sugary foods and the crash that inevitably follows.

The bad news is, once a neural pathway is formed, it's there for life (which is why you never forget how to ride a bicycle, regardless of how little time you spend on two wheels). But the good news is that you can weaken the old, not so good habits by *consciously* choosing to form new, beneficial habits in their place. So what was once a fully-fledged, unhealthy 'road' (habit) in your brain, can now become more of an overgrown dirt track that you don't visit very often! All you have to do is make a new healthier 'road', or habit instead. Remember, one at a time.

SO HOW DO YOU FORM A GOOD HABIT?

Helpful habits are created in exactly the same way as bad habits – **through repetition**. Again, the habit can be imbedded more quickly and more strongly when repetition is combined with emotion.

Most habits are installed unconsciously, without you being aware of what you're doing. But you can also create a new habit deliberately and consciously. Once you understand this, you can install a helpful new habit whenever you're prepared to make the effort.

These beneficial new habits will take you in the direction in which you want to go, rather than sabotaging you, as your bad habits do.

Be aware that building a new habit doesn't happen overnight but if you vividly visualise what you want to achieve (remember the carrot motivation?) and attach a positive emotion such as love, anticipation, pleasure or excitement to it, you'll get there faster and the habit will be deeper.

To keep from sliding back into bad old habits, you have to constantly reinforce helpful new habits by practising them regularly, with energy and emotion. You need to really want the healthier, more helpful outcome and you need to commit to making the good habit your new reality if that is what you really want.

TASK: Decide on a simple new habit that you'd like to form. It could be something like swapping chocolate for fruit, drinking more water, or going for a walk each morning before you start work.

- Plan the actions that you'll need to perform in order to establish the habit.
- Timetable those actions – do them at least once a day, if possible.

- Each morning, set a strong commitment to behave as if you already have the healthy new habit.
- Look forward to your daily practice, even if it feels like an effort at times. Make believe that you're excited by the activity and that you enjoy practising it.
- Keep a journal and note down your attitude to the new activity changes over the coming days and weeks. Also, keep track of the benefits you experience.
- Keep practising the behaviour, even when you don't feel like doing it.

Within weeks, there will come a point where you don't have to make yourself do it anymore. Your mind and body will automatically factor it into your day."

HOW STRESSFUL IS YOUR LIFESTYLE?

Stress is not an imaginary feeling or state of mind. It can be measured, and it can be dangerous to your health. When you are feeling stressed out, the hormones adrenalin and cortisol are released into the bloodstream. Having consistently high levels of cortisol in your blood can lead to numerous health problems including weight gain. This is because cortisol increases your blood sugar level, so any excess glucose that hasn't been used in a stressful event can be stored as fat.

Not only that, some experts estimate that for every year of continued stress, you age by six years! So, reduce your stress levels and keep yourself feeling younger!

"Imagine you have a piggy bank, but instead of money it holds your emotional energy. It's so easy to give give give to people, support them and be there for them, but unless we take time to care for ourselves as well, we start becoming exhausted, overwhelmed and stressed. Our proverbial banks become empty! Keep a balance, and keep your emotional piggy bank topped up!" Jane Travis – Female Psychologist

TIPS FOR MANAGING STRESS AND KEEPING STRESS LEVELS TO A MINIMUM.

- Five-minute meditation – if something winds you up, take five minutes to yourself to breathe

Size HH

deeply and think clearly and calmly.

- If you feel like things are getting too much at times, don't be afraid to talk to someone or ask for help, whether it be with the housework, the kids, or even at work.
- Identify the main stress causes in your life so you can look at each one individually and see what changes can be made.
- Go for what makes your heart truly happy.
- If you are a caregiver of any kind, always be sure to look after yourself as well so that you will be fit and well to look after others.
- If it's someone else making you feel at your wits end, smile, bless them and wish them a good day. If they have a good day, at least they will leave you alone. Remember you never know what other people are going through, or have gone through either. By wishing only positive thoughts towards people that leave you feeling crazed, you have done your bit, and it feels far better than becoming angry.
- Have a good night's rest!

SLEEP

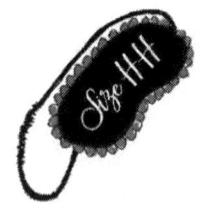

In an ideal world, we would get as much sleep as we needed every night, but in the real world it is not always possible with kids, work and fast paced lifestyles.

Lack of sleep affects pretty much every function of our bodies and minds, so it's definitely worth making it a priority if you don't already. First of all, let's look at why sleep is so important for our wellbeing, then we can look at how to get more much-needed rest.

Sleep helps to regulate the hormones responsible for controlling and affecting your appetite. When you don't get enough sleep, hormones can become imbalanced leading to an increase in appetite. Sleep can also directly affect blood sugar levels and the way our bodies handle insulin.

Size HH

Most of us tend to feel grouchy without enough sleep. This is because cortisol, one of the stress hormones, is usually regulated while you doze away. Without enough quality sleep, your cortisol levels can be unbalanced and become too high. This usually results in mood swings, irritability and generally feeling awful. Good sleep = instant mood boost!

The average adult needs between 7 – 9 hours' sleep per night, but not many of us manage this often enough. A good way to combat fatigue is to take a 20-30-minute siesta or power nap during the day whenever you can, especially if you are planning a late night. If you have kids, sleep when they do (never mind the housework it's not that important), or have a friend or family member watch them for an hour or two while you rest.

Here are a few **tips from The Sleep Guru** that can help you enjoy a more restful night's sleep:

1. **Disconnect yourself from the internet and reconnect to yourself**. When you become disconnected from yourself, you become stressed. Switch off your computer and TV at least 2 hours before bedtime and spend that time reading, taking a hot bath, or anything something else you find relaxing.

2. **Try 30 minutes of deep breathing when you are ready for bed**. *"Learning to make space for the breath is fundamental to health. The heart, mind and breath are intimately connected. Our daily practice should open our heart, calm the mind and lengthen and expand the breath. If we can do that, we open the door to managing stress, reacting less and sleeping well" Anandi*

The moment you bring your attention to your breathing, the breath will lengthen and slow down, your heart rate will slow down, and you will start to feel sleepy. Honestly, it works! Simply lie on your bed, put your hands on your stomach and stay focused on calmly breathing in and out.

3. **Eat at least 2 hours before bed and make it light**

Your evening meal should ideally be something light and easily digested. No heavy lasagne, or rump steak please; have those at lunch! Otherwise, your system will remain busy trying to digest it all, and that's like trying to sleep while you're running a race!

4. **De-clutter your bedroom**

These days, bedrooms are filled with all sorts of junk and clutter. Don't even mention all the rubbish we shove under our beds! Take a little time to pull everything out and get rid of as much as possible. If you have a TV or computer in your bedroom, evict it! Try to make your bedroom an oasis of calm so that as soon as you step through the door, you leave your stress behind you!

5. Make time in your day for you

Bring your life into balance. Running in the fast lane from seven in the morning to nine at night (or sometimes longer!) is not at all balanced. Make the required changes so you have time to slow down before bedtime. Sooner or later, you will be forced to, so better to make the choice now.

THINGS TO AVOID BEFORE BED

Help your body fall into a deeper slumber by avoiding things like caffeine, alcohol, fatty foods and heavily spiced dishes before bed. All of these things, along with focusing on stuff that may be worrying you, have been proven to disrupt sleep. Always try to go to sleep thinking about something happy, no matter what your circumstances, for a more restful night.

Now you can see why sleep should be a priority if you don't want your body to age faster, or suffer from the effects of burning the candle at both ends!

Of course, there will be times where you don't get as much rest as you need. If I wake up in a hideous mood due to lack of sleep, or whatever reason, the last thing I want to do is put on a cheerful exercise DVD and start leaping around the living room. In a tired frame of mind, the only thing I want is coffee and my bed!

Within 10 seconds of opening your eyes, your lifestyle and ingrained habits kick in, making it easier to carry on in the same old way and not making any changes. So, if you do wake up tired and fear your lifestyle is taking over the day again, remember this – even the tiniest effort towards being healthier is <u>always</u> better than nothing!

> *'One positive thought in the morning can change your whole day'. Zig Ziglar*

Size HH

Mindset Trainer Caroline Ferguson offers this tip:

"Every morning, before you put a foot on the floor, set your intention for how you're going to approach the day. Try something like "I can't wait to nourish myself with some delicious, healthy food today!" Remember that your unconscious mind pays attention to emotions, so set your intention with energy and passion and a big smile on your face. Then bounce out of bed and live that intention."

GRATITUDE

Perk yourself up by thinking about something you have to be thankful for, even if it is just for opening your eyes and being able to get out of bed. Be genuinely thankful for it, feel happy about it, then go about your daily business knowing that nothing can take a smile off your face unless you let it. This will take approximately 30 seconds out of your morning. Everyone has time for that and everyone has things to be grateful for!

I'M ON A ROLL BABY!

Maintaining these good efforts is what most consider the hardest part. In fact, the pressure of trying not to fail at this 'healthy eating' malarkey can be a stress factor in itself and actually make things worse. Remember if your motivation is a 'carrot' goal, (meaning you are working towards something with positive emotion, rather than trying to get away from your current state which usually brings a negative emotion) you are far more likely to continue making more and more healthier habits and diminishing the old ones.

Accept that you can't make loads of new habits overnight and if you happen to slip back to an old one, it is not the end of the world - you can choose to re-embrace your new healthy habit whenever you want, even the same day!

Don't delay looking after yourself because your friend's birthday do is next week, do it right now and have a blast at the party! If you are looking after yourself most of the time, then treats are there to be enjoyed. It doesn't mean you have failed because you indulged in a 'not so good' habit. It means tomorrow is a new day, if you are lucky enough to see it, then do something good for your body to say thank you for all it does for you!

Size HH

If you need motivation, re-read the 'Points to Remember' pages in this book to help put you back on track. Sometimes it's good to refresh.

Ask yourself why do you think you go back to old habits? Have you made suitable new ones in their place? Remember you are the one in control.

FOOD IN THE FAST LANE

Back in my days as a care worker, the last thing I was interested in after finishing a night shift was preparing a healthy meal. I just wanted something quick and tasty before hitting the pillows. That was my lifestyle day in day out. Many of you may be in the same situation, possibly even going without food most of the day until the mother of all pig outs during the evening. You are not alone.

It's at times like this when you need to look after yourself most. My body was crying out for protein, vitamins and good fats. I was left feeling tired and emotional with a dull complexion. Shop bought ready meals are not the answer! While they have their place as a quick, occasional option, most of them are high in salt and preservatives as well as nutritionally deficient so shouldn't regularly be eaten or relied upon for nourishment.

If you like ready meals, bulk up on homemade meals and portion some up in the freezer. If you are thinking 'I can't cook, or I don't have the time' you *can* learn to cook your favourite meals. There are heaps of quick, easy-to-make, healthy recipes waiting for you to discover, such as Jamie Oliver's 15 and 30-minute meals. Prioritise that small amount of time to eat and treat yourself well. You are worth the effort!

Failing that, there are some great companies out there that can deliver fresh, healthy food to your home/office, so there are great options for everyone. Eating well gives you the energy and the nutrients your body needs to function at best, greatly reducing the chance of a long list of illnesses.

We all love a takeaway or some fast food now and then, but that's exactly what it should be, now and then. Same as the fizzy drinks you may have with them.

EATING HEALTHILY ON A BUDGET

Some may argue that it is too expensive to buy healthy

foods like fresh organic fruit and veg, meat, etc. While convenience foods may seem like a cheaper, easier option, most people don't realise the amount of money they do spend on things that are essentially making them overweight and unhealthy.

Things like chocolate, energy drinks, crisps, ready meals, etc might only cost a pound or two, but so do apples, bananas, vegetables, meat or fish. If you have a garden, why not try growing some herbs or fruit and veg? If there is a local market or farmers market near you each week, check it out if you have time, there are some amazing fresh food bargains to be found! If you are ready to be Size Happy and Healthy, it may be necessary to make a couple of changes to the things you shop for.

TRY THIS

To begin with, keep the receipts for everything you spend on things that end up in your body, including drinks, alcohol, meals, snacks, everything… At the end of the week, check out your stash! You may be very surprised at how much it costs you, regarding not just your health, but your pocket too.

ALCOHOL

Sorry to sound like a fun spoiler but, alcohol is pretty much just liquid calories. If your lifestyle means that you like to enjoy a drink regularly, just remember it could be a reason you struggle to lose excess body fat. If you don't fancy cutting it out of your life altogether, aim for no more than 1-2 per day and choose some of the 'healthier' options such as red wine, gin and slim tonic with lemon/lime, or half a beer, rather than the sugary cocktails, premade alcopop bottles, or spirits mixed with cola's and fizzy drinks.

HOW ACTIVE ARE YOU?

If you consider yourself active already but still have weight to shift or areas to tone up, this can be helped with what you eat to begin with, followed by targeted exercises. No matter what lifestyle you have, there are ways to fit in more exercise without disrupting your life. Every little helps! Every step counts! I'll give you lots of juicy tips on how to increase your fitness in the exercise section.

Size HH
ARE GOALS OVER-RATED?

Time rolls around quickly so goals can help you to stay on track. If you work well with something to aim at (many people do), think of your motivation and set yourself a "Carrot" goal to help you reach it. Such as the dress you would like to fit in, or a mountain you would like to be fit enough to climb, or a charity race you would like to take part in. Daily goals can be helpful too. For example, to walk 8000 or 10,000 steps per day. (step trackers are a great way to record this).

The next sections of the book are full of nutrition and exercise tips that you can easily fit into any lifestyle, any schedule, whatever mood you wake up in and whatever the day ahead has in store for you.

LIFESTYLE POINTS TO REMEMBER

- Take photos and measurements if you want to track your progress from now
- However busy your schedule, <u>you can</u> become Size Happy and Healthy
- Replace old bad habits with new ones that make you feel amazing instead. Recognise which habits may be keeping you from Size

HH and replace them one by one.
- Stressful lifestyles are not good for the health. Period. If you lead a stressful lifestyle but thrive off being busy, remember busy and stressful are two different things, so be sure to give yourself some wind-down time too!
- Ready meals, packet pasta and noodles, etc are not the answer for regular use. Bulk up on home-made dishes to store in fridge/freezer for easy meals when you need them
- Sleep is an underestimated part of weight loss and wellbeing. Make it a priority and follow our sleep tips
- If you wake up tired, think something positive before you get out of bed and be thankful for it as you start your morning. Then you can begin the day feeling motivated
- If you find your energy flagging during the day, either take a power nap or schedule an early night!
- Whatever your budget, you can afford to be healthy. After analysing how much you spend on things that could essentially make you ill, (takeaways are not cheap), make it a priority

from now on to buy the healthy fuel foods your body needs at the supermarket or local market. If you have everything your body needs, a treat here and there will do no harm, but you must meet your nutritional needs first!
- If you enjoy alcohol, just keep in mind this also adds on to your calorie intake for the day just like a chocolate bar would. Not to mention any other possible side effects…
- Become aware of how much exercise you do without realising and challenge yourself to add to that where you can (everyone can, I will show you how to in the exercise section). Small changes lead to big changes!
- Set yourself goals – Start small, aim high!

Eva George

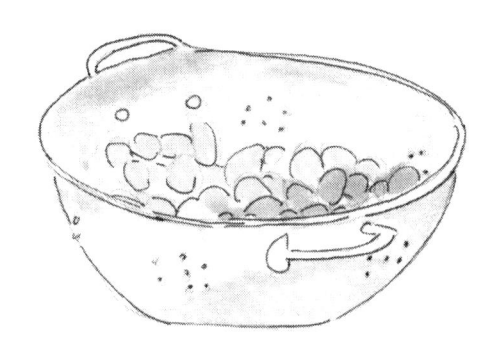

NUTRITION – A GOOD BODY IS MADE IN THE KITCHEN

There are literally thousands of weight-loss diets out there (you may have tried half of them already!) and some of them may work to lose weight. What they don't usually do is work for life, or give your body what it really needs. Some of the 'weight' lost may not necessarily be body fat either, but muscle or water instead. Unless you want to spend your whole life on a diet, there must be a better way to stay in shape, or lose any unhealthy body fat right!? Right.

Girls, women, all females, we are like superwomen (really) and the food we eat is like the fuel we need for our superwoman role. Understanding what fuels our body needs and keeping ourselves topped up regularly is **the key** to Size Happy and Healthy. This will also help to stop a number of unhealthy habits and vicious circles. You won't crave the same things anymore, your tastes buds may even change, and **you will feel satisfied, energetic, healthier** and more confident.

Let's get straight down to business. Everything we share with you is going to be as simple as possible, and I promise not to overload you with jibber jabber and irrelevant information. Our aim is to put a few myths to bed and give you the essential tips you need to make your body thrive.

We don't need to follow the latest diets, we don't need weight-loss pills, and we certainly don't need to spend our precious time aiming for society's perfect size. We need to make the **most of what we have** and this is where to start.

FIND YOUR BALANCE

So what do our bodies really need? Our lifestyle and how active we are must be taken into account before working out what foods we need. Tastes, allergies, cultures, budgets and beliefs all affect the way we eat too, possibly making it seem like too big a challenge to even begin making any changes. That's why we believe in starting with small changes that you can begin with right away.

If the meal on our plate is not a good balance of nutrients, we won't feel satisfied after meals and are more likely to reach for sugary snacks or the wrong types of carbs. Finding the **right balance for you** will help you shed unwanted body fat *healthily* and leave you feeling more energised, satisfied and happier in yourself. Results of exercise will also show up quicker and last longer with the right balance of fuels.

There are six basic nutrients that we can't live without; water, carbohydrates, protein, fat, fibre, vitamins and minerals.

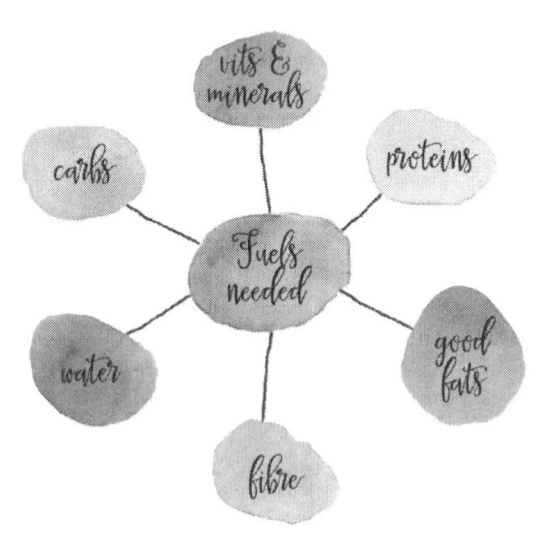

Diagram: "Fuels needed" surrounded by vits & minerals, proteins, good fats, fibre, water, carbs

All of the nutrients above need to be washed down with plenty of water, so let's start there…

WATER – YOUR NEW BEST FRIEND

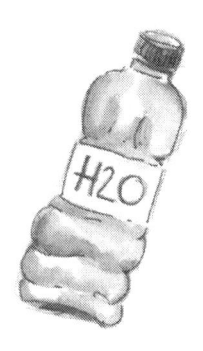

Water contains no calories, fat, or cholesterol and is low in sodium (salt). It is nature's appetite suppressant, hydrator and it helps the body to metabolize fat. It will make your skin glow and keep your systems running as smooth as possible. Need more reasons to drink more water? Ok…

How many times have you headed for the fridge or biscuit tin when you have felt hungry? What if I told you that instead of hunger this is possibly thirst? Next time you find yourself heading in that direction, hold your horses and swiftly pour yourself a drink of water first to find out if you are genuinely hungry, or just thirsty!

Do a quick thirst check now before you read any further…

Feeling thirsty means your body is already dehydrated and needs water, so be sure to sip regularly from now on (before you feel thirsty) to avoid rapid skin aging and other problems. Just a 2% loss of bodyweight in water will cause you problems and a loss of just 5% can be fatal. We lose water constantly through breathing, sweating and urinating, so our entire body relies upon you to give it the water it needs regularly.

Another way to check if you are slightly dehydrated, take a look at the colour of your urine next time you go to the toilet. The darker it is the more dehydrated you are.

Some drinks including coffee, tea, alcohol, many soft drinks and even some sports drinks are known as diuretics, which means they can leave you even more dehydrated as they make you need to use the toilet more frequently. Water really is the healthiest way to stay hydrated, but any fluid is better than nothing.

How much do we need? Ideally at least two litres every day and more if you are exercising or spending time in the sun.

Size HH

It may help to have a 1-litre bottle so you can measure how much you are drinking and aim for two of those per day (more if you are exercising). Until I started measuring, I had no idea how little water I was drinking every day! I had always thought I drank quite a lot!

If you really can't stand plain water, try adding fresh fruit like strawberries, raspberries, blueberries, cucumber, lemon, lime, or a dash of fruit juice.

Natural herbal teas such as fennel or chamomile are great alternatives too; different herbal blends provide different benefits.

DOES GREEN TEA REALLY HELP TO LOSE WEIGHT?

Unfortunately, despite the regular claims, there is no scientific proof that drinking green tea directly helps with weight loss. However, a cup of green tea or similar is obviously the healthier option compared to sugar laden lattes, mochachinos and other popular hot drinks with added sugars.

Anyway, after just a week or two of drinking more water, you will stop needing to run to the ladies room so often (hurrah). Your body will stop flushing and start lapping up the water for all the cells and tissues, resulting in more glowing skin, more of a controlled appetite, and loads more health and beauty benefits!

IS DETOXING JUST ANOTHER FAD DIET?

Our beautiful bodies come with a natural detox system built in as standard! Toxins and waste are released all the time through the lungs, kidneys, liver, bowels and skin. All we have to do is aid that process.

Toxins sneak into the body in many ways, including food, air and synthetic personal care products. If we overload on toxins, some of them can end up being stored in our fat cells along with fat, causing inflammation. The more toxins you have in your body and fat cells, the harder it is to lose weight and the unhealthier you will feel.

Size HH

Here are just a few examples of foods that will aid your body's natural detox process along with water;

Blueberries
Lemon
Red grapes
Cherries
Oranges
Limes
Kiwi fruit
Dark chocolate
Spinach & kale
Wheatgrass
Garlic

Before we look at any more great foods to eat, let's quickly take a look at *how* we eat, as that can make a big difference to a happy and healthy body.

THIS WOULDN'T FEED A RABBIT!

When you're hungry, do you find yourself reaching for a huge portion of your favourite foods? To begin with, try not to let yourself get so hungry (and/or thirsty) in the first place, so wouldn't feel the need to choose a supersize portion. Truth be known, we could eat all of our favourite foods, if we had them in moderation and in balance with the other nutrients we need. If there is a big portion on your plate, you will be likely to eat more, so start with a modest portion and go from there. Using smaller plates is an easy way to do this.

THE 20 MINUTE RULE

20 minutes before you are going to eat, try drinking a glass of tepid water (not cold). This will create a sense of fullness, or at least take the edge off feeling ravenous!

Once you have eaten your meal, drink more water. Then wait 20 minutes before deciding whether you need a second portion. The water will help digest the meal and the 20 minutes is the time needed for our stomach to let your brain know it has just been fed!

So, for roughly 20 minutes after your meal, keep yourself busy; tidy up, prepare dessert, even go for a gentle walk round the block, whatever suits you, just stay busy for 20 minutes to give your body a chance to do its thing. Last of all, always be thankful for the meal you just had, it's more than some people have.

BITE ME!

Becoming aware of chewing means becoming aware of eating and appreciating all of the flavours, rather than mindlessly wolfing down our snacks and dinners. Eating your dinner at 90 miles per hour because you feel famished means you will be more likely to pick afterwards and even go for a second portion – especially if your dinner wasn't sufficiently nutritious to start with.

The more digested the food is when it hits your stomach, the more nutrients our bodies are able to take from it. This is why the new super blenders have become popular. They blend the food to a digested state before we consume them, making it easier for our body to take in as much nutrients as possible. Enjoying a smoothie or juice every day is an easy way of contributing to your vitamin and mineral requirements and eating more whole, raw vegetables, fruit, nuts and seeds.

GIVE IT TO ME RAW!

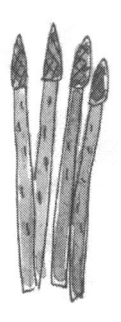

Eating raw food has taken off in the past few years too, with many raw food experts helping us to reap the benefits of not cooking food. They say that cooking kills vital nutrients, which it will, if you over fry or boil the life out of your food. It's back to having balance again. Try adding a few raw meals and snacks as often as you can for an instant nutrition boost (even if it is just an apple or a few sticks of celery and hummus, it still counts!). Take it slowly though as your body may not be used to raw.

Size HH
COOKED FOOD LOVERS

The way foods are cooked and prepared can influence how healthy they are. Cooking certain carbohydrates makes them absorbed by the body quicker, giving a fast insulin release (the same effect as sugar to the body, only better for you). For instance, boiled potatoes are more steadily absorbed by the body than baked or microwaved potatoes, so boiled would be a healthier option.

For the healthiest way to cook, try to either; bake, grill, poach, or steam foods wherever possible rather than microwave, fry or over-boil.

BREAKFAST

We are bombarded with conflicting studies about whether having breakfast makes a difference to the metabolism and losing weight. The truth is everyone is different, and our unique lifestyles can mean that breakfast may not be the traditional 7/8am sit down. Not everyone fancies breakfast when they first wake up either. If you are really not a breakfast person, at least make sure you **drink** water within an hour of waking, **(or fresh lemon water if possible)**.

Rehydrating after sleep is essential (don't get me started on the whole water subject again!).

However, **it is extremely beneficial to have breakfast,** whatever time that happens to be, because it provides the energy you need for the hours ahead, as well as waking up the digestive system and metabolism. Breakfast can also help you EAT LESS later in the evening by filling you up earlier on.

What is good for breakfast? Try different things to see what suits you and your lifestyle. Obviously the healthier you make it, the better off you will be. Things like, eggs and salmon or porridge with berries have loads of goodness and fill you up all morning. Good quality meal replacement shakes or protein-rich smoothies are an option if you don't have much time, or don't fancy physical food first thing in the morning. Just be sure to do your research into which brand you go for.

~ Eating well is a form of self-respect ~

Size HH
EAT AND LOSE?

Have you heard the theory about eating five to six times per day to lose weight quicker? Unfortunately, just by eating six meals per day, you metabolism won't suddenly jumpstart into more calorie burning, however, it can help to sustain energy, as can healthy snacks.

Unless you are muscle building, or already used to a regular eating routine, aiming for six healthy meals per day could probably just complicate things for you (or not, everyone is different). However, by making breakfast, lunch and dinner into three **habitual** meals every day, your brain will have to make much fewer decisions based on willpower and will know exactly what it's doing. Breakfast, lunch and dinner. Simple!

Even preparing your meals (in your head, or on paper) the night before can make new healthy habits easier by already deciding what you will be doing for those three meals the next day. You could go one step further and actually prepare some, or all three your meals for the next day and put in the fridge ready, or at least have the ingredients ready. That way you have some kind of plan, leaving fewer decisions to will power which is constantly zapped by making decisions on other things. Keep it simple for yourself with three scrumptious meals that you look forward to.

Picking on little things all day then a huge meal at night won't do you many favours either. If this sounds like you, it is important to find ways to plan your three meals per day and eat well at each one of them. If you still find yourself with the 4 pm munchies, first drink water, then check the time to see how long until dinner, if you really can't wait, try to go for something with benefits *other* than just tasting good. Fruit is always a quick, tasty option and rich in fuels to give you energy.

WHY WE NEED CARBS IN OUR LIFE!

We have all heard about a no carb, or low carb diet. This type of dieting involves cutting out foods like rice, pasta, baked goods, pizza, breads etc in a bid to lose weight or body fat. Cutting back on certain types of carbohydrates can help with weight loss because it is these types of foods that can easily tip the balance in favour of fat storage (you know the types, donuts, muffins, fries etc.).

When we overload on carbs without burning enough off as energy (through activity), the body stores it as fat for energy later on. Excess consumption of carbohydrates over time can also lead to depression and serious diseases like cancer and diabetes.

It wouldn't make sense to cut out all carbs though! Neither would you want to, carbohydrates are one of your body's main source of energy and are important for several health reasons.

WHAT ARE CARBS?

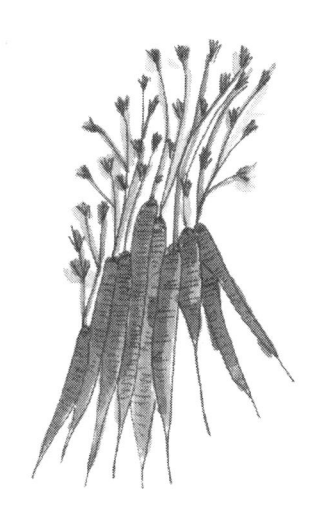

There are three different types of carbohydrates:

- Sugar (natural or artificial) is found in things like jams and condiments, soft drinks and juices, fruit, many breakfast cereals and all the other sweet stuff we know about. It is fast digesting and provides a quick burst of energy. More about sugar later.
- Starch is made up of many natural sugar (glucose) units bonded together and is found in food that comes from plants such as potatoes, corn, pumpkin, peas, beans and lentils. Starchy foods provide a slow, steady release of energy throughout the day.
- Fibre is only found in foods that come from plants. It doesn't provide an energy boost directly, but it does help eliminate waste build up that causes fatigue, so it can help with energy levels. More on fibre shortly...

Size HH

THE HEALTHIEST TYPES OF CARBS

Breads – Wholegrain, bran, rye, and sourdough bread
Wholegrain rice
Whole wheat pasta
Rice noodles
Wholegrain cereals without sugar
Peas, lentils, red kidney beans, chickpeas
Cous cous
Oats
Quinoa
Buckwheat
Fresh fruit such as peaches, apples, pears, cherries, coconut, plums, grapefruit, grapes, banana
Fresh fruit juice (not concentrated and with no added sugar)
Yoghurts with no added sugars or sweeteners
Dark chocolate (over 60% cocoa)
Soya products (if no allergies)
Vegetables including tomatoes (yes I know technically a fruit), mushrooms, carrots, broccoli, cabbage, kale, cauliflower, fresh corn.
Honey

When you think of carbs from now on, think of these lot above!

WHAT'S THE DEAL AND HOW MUCH IS TOO MUCH?

- Carbs like pastas, rice, potatoes etc should be a portion roughly the size of your fist so you don't tip the balance
- Go for the wholegrain and whole meal varieties of breads, pastas and rice whenever possible unless you have allergies to gluten, then go for gluten free varieties
- If you are having potatoes, wash well and keep the skins on for more nutrition
- Aim for at least 5 portions of fruit and vegetables per day for your carbohydrate *and* vitamin requirements.
- Frozen fruit and vegetables can be useful to stock up on. They are usually frozen quickly from fresh so could have higher nutrition content than fruit which has been shipped around and sat in supermarkets. Plus, it lasts longer and makes easy work of amazing smoothies!

Size HH

FIBRE

Ok so not the prettiest subject to talk about, but essential for becoming Size HH! Fibre keeps us feeling fuller and more satisfied for longer. There are two types of fibre, soluble (can be digested) and insoluble (cannot be digested).

By eating a variety of fruit, vegetables and wholegrains **every day**, you should have enough of both types. If you don't eat much fibre at the moment, it's important not to rush off and stuff yourself with loads in a bid to 'cleanse' as this will only result in bloating and wind! Definitely not what we want, so start with small changes such as:

- Leaving the skins on potatoes, veg and fruits where possible
- Having porridge and/or fruit for breakfast instead of a muffin, or sugary cereal
- Eating more fresh fruit and vegetables everyday

FIBRE RICH FOODS OUR BODY WOULD LOVE US TO EAT REGULARLY;

- Oats, barley and rye
- Fruit, such as apples (skin on), figs, ripe bananas, avocado, raspberries, blackberries, pears, mango, guava
- Vegetables, such as carrots and potatoes (skins on), artichoke, peas, broccoli,
- Wholegrain bread/whole meal rolls
- Bran/cereals
- Nuts, seeds (chia are great), beans, lentils and pulses (especially flaxseeds! Flax contain a large amount of fibre making it an ideal tool to aid your body's natural detox process. Only use ground flaxseeds though as the whole seeds just pass through the digestive system and we take nothing from it).

Most importantly, fibre needs water to do its job properly!

Size HH

HOW MUCH FIBRE SHOULD WE AIM FOR?

Each of us has a slightly different requirement for fibre, but UK NHS guidelines say to aim for at least 30 grams per day.

If you have IBS, it is important to talk to your doctor about your fibre intake and how much you need.

PROBIOTICS DRINKS, DO THEY MAKE ANY DIFFERENCE?

Without going too scientific on you all, probiotics are said to help aid digestion and detoxification by supporting stomach and bowel health. Probiotics are the naturally occurring good bacteria in the gut. The balance of good and bad bacteria in the gut can be affected by diet, pollution and high cortisol levels (one of the stress hormones). Tummy health is extremely important for becoming the best version of you. It leads to more energy and a better mood. People with an unhealthy gut may find it very hard to lose excess body fat and may frequently find themselves with low mood and energy levels. If you can remember to take a low sugar probiotic drink when you wake up every morning, before tea/coffee, you will be doing your digestive system a little favour.

PROTEIN

If you can include protein in every meal or snack, you are onto a winner! Our bodies, skin, hair, nails, muscles, are all made from protein and so it's essential for recovery and encouraging fresh, new cell growth. Our bodies cannot store it either, so it's essential that we top it up regularly.

HOW PROTEIN AFFECTS WELLBEING, WEIGHT, AND BODY FAT LEVELS;

- Helps to maintain and support muscle mass (essential for toning up)
- Stops cravings
- Leaves us feeling full and satisfied
- Look healthier (new skin cells are made from protein)
- Feel stronger (your muscles will love you for it)

Size HH
ANIMAL AND PLANT PROTEINS

Protein doesn't necessarily mean meat; there are plenty of vegetarian and vegan options available too. All animal and plant cells contain some protein, but the amount of protein present in food varies widely. Vegetarians need to think about this carefully about where they will get their protein from so that they can maintain a balanced diet.

Let's take a look at the different types, any time you need some food inspiration, remember these:

FOR NON VEGGIES
MEAT AND POULTRY;
- Chicken breast (skinless)
- Turkey breast (skinless)
- Very lean cuts of beef
- Lean bacon (grilled not fried)
- Lamb/Pork chops

FISH AND SEAFOOD
- Sardines
- Tuna
- Sea Bass
- Shrimp
- Clams

- Lobster
- Cod
- Crab meat
- Salmon
- Calamari
- Haddock

DAIRY

- Milk – (many versions available including lactose-free, raw and organic)
- Yoghurts – Natural, unsweetened yoghurts are great little snack and a quick source of protein
- Cheese - (made with cow, goat, or sheep's milk) In small amounts, certain cheeses such as organic cheese, cottage cheese, vintage cheddar and ricotta can be nutritionally beneficial and very satisfying! It can be an easy way of contributing to our protein and calcium requirements. Sprinkle of parmesan? Cheese and wine night? Too right!
- Butter and margarine - Try to swap margarine for butter where possible, even using nut and seed butter as delicious, healthier alternatives.

Size HH

NUTS, PULSES AND SEEDS

- Almonds, unsalted cashews and peanuts, pistachios
- Lentils, pumpkin seeds, sunflower, flaxseeds, sesame seeds and watermelon.
- Beans - soy beans, kidney beans, black beans, white beans, dry roasted soy beans and lima beans

VEGETABLES

- Broccoli
- Spinach
- Kale
- Artichoke
- Corn
- Brussel sprouts
- Bean sprouts
- Potatoes (with skin on) and sweet potatoes
- Fruit (not generally thought of as a protein source but some contain more than others)
- Grapefruit, blackberries, watermelon, orange, banana, dates, prunes, guava, avocado, raspberries, peaches, figs, grapefruit, cantaloupe, apricots, strawberries, pomegranate

OTHER PROTEIN SOURCES

- Eggs
- Marmite
- Protein shakes
- Tofu (Soy)
- Sietan
- Whey

HOW MUCH PROTEIN DO YOU NEED DAILY?

There is no exact amount given as an official recommendation for protein as it really depends on various factors including; your weight, your age and your current exercise levels. Just by including a variety of proteins (like these above) in your meals and snacks every day you should getting a good enough balance.

WHO ARE YOU CALLING FAT?

When some people think about slimming down, they think cutting down on fat is the way forward. Even going as far as buying only low-fat, or fat-free meal options and wondering why they start feeling glum and not losing any weight. Keep in mind, the label may say low fat but it may be high in sugar and/or salt. Women, in particular, *need* certain fats, in small doses.

Fat is the most concentrated source of stored energy in our bodies and is necessary for a variety of roles including; making hormones including oestrogen and for the absorption of vitamins A, D and E. Good fats also helps to give our skin and hair a healthy glow.

With so many mixed messages about fats, it's hard to know what is best. If we are aiming to be healthier, then fats like those found in cream, chocolate and fatty cuts of red meat, are the types we wouldn't want to eat every single day if we were aiming for optimum health. With that in mind, let's take a look at the kind of foods we *should* be taking our fat requirements from.

GOOD FATS CAN BE FOUND IN;
- Oily Fish – Sardines, mackerel, salmon, herring, trout
- Nuts – walnuts, peanuts, cashews, hazelnuts, pecans, macadamias
- Seeds - Sunflower, sesame, pumpkin, flax and

chia
- Avocados, olives, eggs, coconut oil (coconut oil is a saturated fat but still holds more nutritional benefits than other saturated fats)

HOW MUCH FAT?

Too much fat, especially saturated fats, in your diet, can lead to serious conditions including heart disease. Saturated fats are hidden in many of the foods and drinks we know and love so for the sake of your health; please keep this information in mind. Guidelines recommend that women should aim for less than 20g of saturated fats per day.

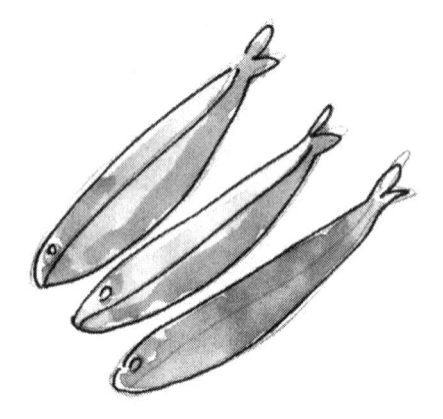

Size HH
OMEGA 3 AND 6S

WHAT ARE THEY?

Omega 3 and 6 are essential fatty acids and only available through food. We need them in small, balanced amounts to be as healthy. Many of us get enough omega 6s through cooking oils, meat and shop bought products containing vegetable oil, but lack the much needed Omega 3's, throwing us out of balance.

Here are ways to bring back the omega balance;

- Use more olive oil instead of vegetable oils (olive oil is rich in good fats and has no effect on insulin which is good news for those with diabetes.) There is no need to fork out on expensive extra virgin oils for cooking though as it can't reach a very high temperature without losing its nutrients. The premium stuff is better saved for salads and dressings.
- Go for grass fed meat and animal products where possible. You may not think it matters but, what they eat, we eat, and grain fed have been shown to be higher in omega 6's and low in omega 3's
- Check the ingredients of your favourite

crackers, pasta sauces, bread etc as vegetable oil lurks in surprising places making you possibly eat more of it than you realise.

- Try to eat oily fish at least once, or twice per week if possible such as sardines, pilchards, salmon, mackerel, anchovies, etc
- Try flaxseed supplements. Ground flaxseeds are high in omega 3 and low in carbohydrates. They can be sprinkled into cereals, yogurts, salads, smoothies and many every day meals and snacks for an extra health boost plus they make you feel fuller for longer! Just when you thought flaxseeds couldn't get any better, they also help to dissolve and eliminate unhealthy fats from the digestive system, so they are not stored as body fat! Well worth the investment.

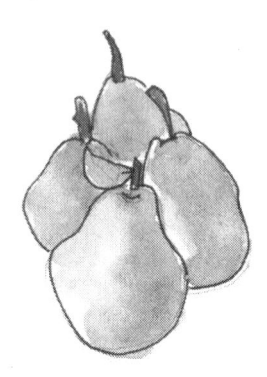

Size HH
SUGAR, SALT AND ALL THINGS HERB AND SPICE

HEY SUGAR

Do you find yourself craving those naughty sweet treats quite often? Sugar affects the feel-good chemicals in the brain, making us crave the same great feelings over and over again. Sugar addiction is a legitimate thing, and you can become hooked as early as childhood.

The frustrating thing is that sugar is everywhere! It is hidden in so many food/drink products and sometimes given confusing names on product labels so that we don't recognise it there (usually ends in 'ose' like glucose, fructose, maltose, lactose, etc). Not surprising so many of us have slowly become addicted to it! Our bodies are not designed to handle the amount of sugar many of us are consuming every day, so instead of being used for energy it has plenty of opportunity to be stored as fat! It also completely messes around with insulin levels, which can easily lead to serious health conditions including diabetes.

Food/drink manufacturers design junk food to keep you coming back for more, it doesn't happen by accident, and it's not your fault! They want us addicted to their products. They don't care about our health.

We are so busy enjoying the sweet taste and the happy feeling we experience while eating, that we ignore the signal from the brain to say we have had enough and just keep going!

Remember, food shopping can easily become a habit, just like anything else. You may be buying the same sweet foods over and over again not just because you like them, and they taste great, but also out of habit. Your brain has probably associated these foods with good times, tastes and feelings, so it becomes a deep, ingrained habit, pushing to have its' own way, like a persistent child.

For instance, your brain may associate a certain time of day, or a TV program, a chair you sit in, or other things, as a trigger for wanting foods you have enjoyed there previously. Remember, once you have become aware of a habit that is not benefitting your health and feel ready to change it, you can start weakening that habit right away, by consciously creating a new one in its' place. By practicing the new healthy habit with positive emotion every day for just a few weeks (as we discussed in the Lifestyle section), you will be able to replace the old bad habit with something that will genuinely make you feel awesome! If you want to that is....

If you are frequently tempted by sweet foods in your fridge and cupboards and would like to have the strength to stop eating them as much, instead of leaving it all up to willpower, make it easier for yourself and don't buy them! Then it won't be *as easy* to snack on them. Try to avoid supermarkets when hungry, it only leads to spending your hard earned cash on the wrong foods.

Sometimes we just fancy something sweet. Any type of fruit, dates, dark chocolate or even yoghurt with honey are great options, as they give nutrition as well as sweetness. Try and make as many healthy swaps like this as you can, because each one will be a boost for your wellbeing!

There are hundreds of healthy sweet snack ideas online to suit all tastes, so I am not going to list anymore here, but I can assure you there are some divine dessert and snack ideas to settle your sweet tooth *and* provide you with health benefits too.

We do need some sugar in our balance, so it is essential not to try and cut it all out, but we could easily have all we need per day from just fruit and dairy alone.

HOW MUCH SUGAR IS OK?

Aim for no more than 25/30g per day (around six teaspoons) ideally made up from all kinds of different sugars, rather than the granulated table sugar you may sling in your coffee. Try to take your sugar requirements from foods that hold other nutrition benefits for you too, rather than the confectionary foods that are constantly 'on offer' at the supermarkets. Otherwise, you are essentially paying to make yourself feel awful and possibly ill.

WISER SUGAR CHOICES;
- Half a teaspoon of honey (raw and locally produced if possible) can be used as a substitute for sugar in tea and coffee. It tastes just as good, and it's a slightly more beneficial alternative.

Size HH

- Maple syrup holds more nutritional benefits than normal sugar and can be used as a sweet substitute for sugar inside birthday cakes and desserts, making it a slightly healthier option for kids too.
- Coconut oil or milk can be used very widely in place of sugar if you want to add few nutritional benefits and a subtle coconut flavour to sweet or savoury dishes.
- Try using sweet berries and currents like blueberries, raspberries, cranberries, and blackberries, etc. instead of sugar on your porridge or Weetabix etc.
- Instead of using shop bought, sugar packed jams with little nutritional value, have a go at making a healthier version using chia seeds and black currants instead of pectin and table sugar! If you need to sweeten it up a little more, you could add a dash of maple, which holds slightly more nutritional benefit than standard granulated sugar.
- Coconut sugar is a slightly better alternative to normal cane sugar as it contains some nutrients. However it is still sugar, so should still be used in moderation.

- Shop bought sweeteners can add the sweetness you require without the sugar or fat, so can be a great option for people with diabetes. Many people are worried about whether sweeteners are bad for our health, but you may find it reassuring to know that all sweeteners in the EU will have been vigorously tested for human consumption. According to Cancer Research UK, there is no evidence linking sweeteners to cancer either, contrary to horror stories may have read on the internet.

SALT

A bit like sugar, the taste of salt can become highly addictive and is hidden in many of the foods we enjoy. Table salt is made from sodium and chloride. We do need sodium, but like everything in this book (and life), it needs a balance.

The national guidelines given in the UK are anything over 2.4g sodium (6g of table salt) per day raises the risk of high blood pressure, which in turn may lead to many other health risks that we want to stay clear of.

Size HH

Going over the recommended daily amount on a daily basis can add up to an unhealthy result. No-one wants a stroke or heart problems.

Of course, none of us are going to start digging the scales out to measure how much salt we eat every day. So, to put it simply, salt is great to be enjoyed as a seasoning as it has done for hundreds of years, just be mindful of what products you eat with salt already in them before adding any more.

Always check product ingredients list, you will be astonished how much salt is used, making it easy to take you over the RDA in just one meal. Some takeaways and fast foods could win medals if the salt content in meals was a competition.

If you know you can be a little 'shake happy' with the salt pot sometimes (possibly out of habit), see if any of these alternatives can work for you instead.

- Wake up your taste buds to new zingy flavours you will learn to appreciate just as much, by adding fresh herbs, spices and peppers to your meals. If buying premixed seasonings, always be sure they have no salt in them and preferably no artificial anything else either!

- Herbs and spices add nutrition to the meal, even if it's a small amount, it still counts!
- Seaweed flakes are an excellent, beneficial alternative to salt and provide a nice taste. Seaweed can be used widely in cooking.
- Balsamic vinegars provide a fantastic zing as do finely chopped onions…ok feeling peckish now!
- Powdered garlic is another good one, again just be sure to pick up the one without salt
- Chilli – some like it hot and it really works to kill off salt cravings…
- Lemon juice – Sharp, tangy and incredibly good for us.
- If you really are a lover of salt and would like the healthiest option, choose the unrefined rock or sea salt (Himalayan pink salt is also a good option). Unrefined means it still contains trace minerals and goodness, so these are the ones to go for. Standard table salt has had all the goodness removed, plus other things added.

Remember we do need sodium, so try to take it from healthy foods instead of processed table salt. The foods below are examples of healthy foods that

Size HH

naturally contain sodium. These are the foods we want to be making our RDA up from.

- Meat/fish
- Veg like; Celery, carrots, sweet potatoes, radish, beetroot, cabbage and cauliflower
- Greens such as; Spinach and swiss chard
- Almonds
- Apricots

VITAMINS AND MINERALS

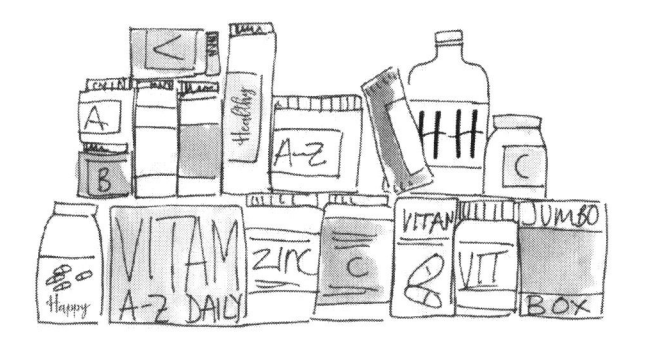

"Ever since my mum was diagnosed with osteoporosis, it has made me more aware of the possible effects of a long term diet lacking in vital vitamins and minerals. Now I make an extra effort to be wise with my food choices and be mindful of how it affects my health and general wellbeing.

I need plenty of energy to keep up with my three active doggies and to be on top form for a job I love, so one of my priorities is to make sure I meet my vitamin and mineral requirements every day. It's never too late, or too early to consciously treat yourself well so you can live your life to the fullest and possibly prevent unnecessary health conditions such as osteoporosis later on." Jacqui Malpass, Editor.

Despite being needed in relatively small amounts, vitamins and minerals are necessary for life and good health. There are 13 vitamins and 22 essential minerals that we need to take from food, water and sunlight.

WHAT ARE VITAMINS?

Vitamins are organic substances that are needed for many actions behind the scenes of our body. Vitamin supplements can be a great way to help you meet your daily requirements and keep your levels topped up continuously, even when you are having an off day. Just remember to consult your doctor before taking any kind of supplements, especially if you are on medication and be sure to stick to correct dosage.

As we age, we require different amounts of vitamins and minerals, depending on our lifestyles, medical conditions, etc. Let's take a look at the main vitamins we need to become Size Happy and Healthy and a few examples of where to find each one:

- **Vitamin A** has important roles in our bodies including helping our immune systems to stay healthy and keeping our skin healthy.
- **Where to find Vitamin A's -** Milk, eggs, oily fish, liver, leafy greens like spinach, sweet potato, carrots, yellow peppers, pumpkin, dried apricots.
- **B Vitamins (B6 and B12)** are important for metabolism and detoxification of certain hormones including cortisol (the stress hormone) and environmental toxins. B Vits also help the body to release the energy we need from carbs and protein.
- **Where to find B vitamins** – Fish, chicken, turkey, chickpeas, wholegrain products, almonds, pecans, dark leafy greens, ham and

added to some breakfast cereals

- **Vitamin C** is another antioxidant, particularly effective at helping with free radical damage caused by smoking and pollution. It is crucial we keep Vitamin C topped up regularly as the body cannot produce it.
- **Where to find Vitamin C** – Red peppers are the richest food in Vitamin C, some other great choices are kiwi fruit, lychee, orange, mango, grapefruit, papaya, pineapple, kale, broccoli, Brussel sprouts, garlic, tomatoes, and wasabi.
- **Vitamin D** should be a hero in the weight-loss world! The right amount helps to slow the production of enzymes that cause the body to store fat and directly helps the metabolism.
- **Where to find Vitamin D** – Sunlight encourages production of vitamin D in the body, so around 20 minutes of fresh air per day can be helpful. Even if it is not sunny outside, as long as it's light, the ultra violet rays will still be present enough to help you produce vitamin D. We can also find this vitamin in foods such as oily fish, meat and eggs.
- **Vitamin E** is the main defender against free

radical damage and is excellent for cell repair. This is why many beauty products contain vitamin E.

- **Where to find it Vitamin E** - Sunflower seeds, spinach, almonds, cashews, hazel nuts, pine nuts, peanuts, tofu, avocado, papaya, prawns, broccoli, red peppers, fresh corn, soya, olives, pumpkin, squash, wheat germ oil, coconut oil, chilli powder, paprika and tomatoes.
- **Vitamin K1 & K2** – These two K vitamins might be in the same group but they have very different roles. K1 is important for blood clotting and K2 is vital for the delivery of calcium from the arteries to the bones where it belongs, as well as assisting vitamins A and D with their jobs.
- **Where to find Vitamin K1 & K2** – K1 is found in green leafy vegetables like broccoli, kale, spinach and K2 can be found in foods like; beef, pork, poultry, egg yolk, dairy, natto (fermented soy beans), sauerkraut (fermented cabbage) organ meats and fish eggs.

For an easy way to cram many vitamins into your meals, try to add as much colour variety as possible.

For example have some from the green range such as peas, lettuce, spinach or broccoli, some from the yellow/orange such as apricot, lemon, sweetcorn or carrots, and some from the red range such as apples, grapes, tomatoes and red peppers. By having *at least* one food from each colour throughout the day, you should find a nice balance.

WHAT ARE MINERALS?
Like vitamins, minerals are substances needed by the body in small amounts for a variety of roles around the body.

Eating a varied diet will ensure an adequate supply of most minerals for healthy people. Some people may require supplements, especially as we age. However it is important to consult your doctor to ensure correct dosage and no interference with other medication.

PARTICULAR MINERALS TO HELP YOU REACH A HAPPY, HEALTHY BODY…
CALCIUM
Calcium is the most abundant mineral in the body.

Most people know it helps build strong bones and teeth, but many don't know it also helps to regulate muscle contractions, including the heart.

Where to find it? Many of us take our calcium from dairy, although other calcium sources can be things like; beans, oily fish, cabbage, Bok choy (Chinese cabbage), broccoli, kale, peas, figs, oranges, tofu, almonds, sesame seeds and oatmeal.

ZINC

Essential for people who want to lose excess body fat. It helps your body to produce the right enzymes needed to digest food properly, especially good for breaking down protein. Zinc also works together with vitamins A and E for healthy thyroid function. Not only that, but zinc also helps with appetite control and immune system!

Where to find it? Lean beef, lamb, turkey, oysters, spinach, pumpkin and sesame seeds, lentils, cashew nuts, dark chocolate, garlic, chickpeas and beans.

MAGNESIUM

To keep it simple, Magnesium encourages better

sleep, helps with flexibility in the muscles, helps to flush toxins through bowels and is essential for proper hydration.

Where to find it? Dark leafy greens like broccoli and peas, nuts and seeds (almonds, cashew, sesame and flax are good examples), fish, avocados, wholegrains, dark chocolate, tofu, natural yoghurt, milk, oats, bananas and dried fruit.

IODINE

This mineral is very helpful for healthy thyroid function (the gland that regulates metabolism). We know that metabolism affects body fat and energy levels.

Where to find it? Eggs, milk, Greek yoghurt, seaweed, cod and other fish.

EATING IN AND DINING OUT

DINING ALONE?

Meals for one can seem like a chore to make the effort with sometimes, especially if we don't have much time. To make things easier and leave fewer decisions to possibly flagging willpower, it may be worth investing an hour to prepare some well-balanced meals for the week, or next few days ahead, then store them in the fridge or freezer, ready for quick, easy reach. Failing to prepare is preparing to fail right?

EATING WITH KIDS?

Setting a good example for the younger generation for eating is obviously essential. If you have kids, every day is a great opportunity to introduce them to the healthiest foods possible, even if they don't eat them at first, just them seeing what you eat will broaden their food knowledge. This can only be a good thing! If you don't already, try to sit down and have your meal when the kids eat, they will enjoy it, and it may save you from eating a meal before bed. As we know, that's not the ideal recipe for a good night's sleep or waistline.

EATING WITH A PARTNER?

Yes sometimes it's easy to get caught up cooking amazing meals, or enjoying take outs together as you settle into loved-up bliss. Then before you know it, you are both thinking you have let yourselves go and don't know where to start. If that sounds like you, take the reins on this one. You can still enjoy great food together, but making small changes to the things you buy and the way you cook and eat, will definitely make a positive difference.

DINING OUT

Life is there to be lived; we don't believe in dieting. If you want to go out and eat what you fancy occasionally, then do it! If you are eating well the rest of the time, who cares if you go for a three course with a slice of something delicious for dessert! When we keep our treat foods to occasions, it makes us appreciate them more, rather than having them every day or very regularly.

A treat does not always have to mean something unhealthy anyway. Go on treat yourself to something that will taste amazing while you eat it *and* help to make you feel and look good afterwards! Take a look at our easy to make raw chocolate recipe from our Editor Jacqui Malpass and loads of other scrumptious recipes on our blog!

TRY THIS

Some people, like our very own Natalie, find it useful

Size HH

to make a food journal or diary, or use an online app to keep track of their food and water intake. Give it a go for one week and see how you get on, let us know what you discover!

If you want to find out more about what you need (or don't need) on a deeper level, a qualified nutritionist could give you a personalised evaluation and assess you for any potential food intolerances or allergies that may be preventing you from Size HH.

NUTRITION POINTS TO REMEMBER

- Aid your natural detox process by drinking water regularly, keeping your body hydrated so it can perform at its best. Water also helps to suppress hunger!
- If you love big portion sizes, try going for smaller plates.
- Finish every meal with a glass of water to wash it down and aid digestion.
- Eat slower and chew well! Sounds basic but it works on so many levels to help us feel full and more satisfied.
- It's a great idea to include raw foods (like fruit and veg) into your daily snacks and meals for

an extra nutrition boost.

- Make an effort to eat and drink something within an hour of waking to start your day in the healthiest way. Things like fruit salad, porridge, yoghurt, eggs (poached, boiled, and scrambled), salmon, wholegrain bread, smoothies made with veg and fruit are all great options if you were wondering.
- If you feel like you hardly eat anything but still can't lose weight, it may be that your body needs assistance with detoxing firstly, followed by regular, healthy fuels for the metabolism. Three balanced meals throughout the day will keep it simple for your mind and body.
- Sometimes snacks are needed to get you through the day. If so, go for something rich in nutrition like vitamins and fibre to aid your natural detox process.
- There is no need to cut carbs from your life; we need them! Just choose some of the 'better for you' carbs to fill up on instead like the types with no added sugars.
- Include some form of protein in every meal or snack for a faster route to Size HH, there are

loads of different options available to suit all tastes.
- Now you know those low-fat options aren't necessarily any better for you, it can save you the bother of looking for them! Good fats, like omega 3's, are the kind of fats we want to include in our meals regularly. Saturated fats and trans fats are the ones that could lead us into health troubles.
- Yep, we need a small amount of sugar in our balance too. Be brave, try some of our wiser sugar choice ideas and let us know how you get on!
- Fibre is absolutely crucial to a happy, healthy body. Find it. Eat it. Say no more!
- Remember salt and sodium are two different things. It is sodium we need and only in small amounts
- When in doubt, get the herbs and spices out! Make even the simplest, healthiest meal taste mouth-wateringly superb with delicious seasonings
- Vitamins are little tiny superheroes! We need them in our lives, every day.
- Don't beat yourself up about nights out, or

falling back to old habits occasionally. If you are looking after yourself most of the time, you deserve a treat!

- If you still find yourself snacking after meals out of habit, try brushing and flossing your teeth. Some people find they are less likely to eat again for a while afterwards.
- Focus on finding and eating foods you know will be amazing for your body and mind. As we have learned, our food intake affects everything, even our mental wellbeing. So, if you find yourself feeling low and you're not quite sure why, firstly consider your thoughts using our tips from the mind section, then take a look at what you have been eating. Maybe starting a food/drink diary to help you.
- Eating good food will make you feel and look good. Fact.
- Everything is about balance!

So, now we know we can still enjoy our favourite things and become healthier, lose excess weight and feel better than ever, by *using* food as your tool to do that. Which nutritious foods will you be choosing today?

Size HH

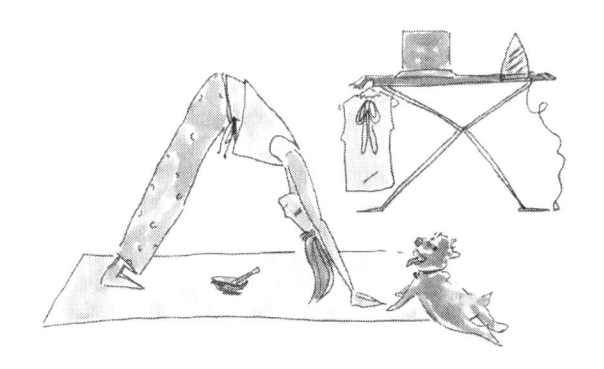

EXERCISE

STRETCHING, POSTURE & TONING

This section is for people who either don't like, or don't have time for the gym, or long workouts. I wanted to show a way forward for those that feel they cannot do traditional exercise for whatever reason, but would like to become fitter health wise, or tone up and lose excess body fat in certain areas.

Many of us become so revved up about a new healthy eating regime and the prospect of feeling fabulous, that we plan up a whole new exercise routine to go along with it. That's what everyone says right? Eat less and do more exercise? Trying to become used to a new eating pattern at the same time as a vigorous new work-out routine is why so many people can't keep it up for long, then feel like they have failed. One habit at a time remember.

Unless you already have a habitual exercise routine set up, the best advice I could give is to make sure your eating habits are right first, then incorporate more and more exercise in as you go along. Meanwhile there are subtle exercises you could start doing today, without disrupting your lifestyle.

Size HH

All movements are a form of exercise. Every movement counts and the more you do the better you will feel for it! This means that you can fit exercise into your routine starting right now and slowly build yourself up to levels you never thought possible!

You could even be exercising your muscles whilst reading this. Just sit up straight, stomach in, clench your bum cheeks and hold for as long as you can, then relax and repeat! Yes, this helps if you do it often!

Even simply standing up requires the use of various muscles to hold us upright. Doesn't sound like much does it and you might be wondering how that could affect your figure or wellbeing, but honestly if you are eating right and do certain little things every day, you WILL see and feel a positive difference, inspiring you to do even more.

If people put as much effort into toning the part of the body they dislike as they do hating it, they would end up looking and feeling utterly amazing!

Eva George

STRETCHING

When you wake up in the morning, the first thing your body wants to do is stretch after being in the same positions for so long, though many of us don't give it the chance. Heaving ourselves out of bed and into our day with the sound of an alarm clock, or a baby crying, or dog wanting attention (insert your scenario here), is all too common for most of us on a regular basis. The thing is, if we all had the time and grace to wake up and practice yoga every morning, we would right? In most people's worlds that is not reality, but everyone still needs to stretch. Without it, the day can seem like hard work before it has even begun!

Stretching our muscles, tendons and ligaments every day, even just a little, helps to prevent our bodies stiffening up and really relieves tension (among other benefits). So even if you are running late, give yourself just a minute to give your body a good stretch, with some deep breaths.

Try starting with what naturally feels good and build yourself up from there. Stretching your muscles can actually feel like a proper workout if you really push yourself, so its' powers are not to be under estimated.

You can begin your warm up for the day before you have even clambered out of bed!

If you need some stretch inspiration try these really simple moves for example. They take less than five minutes and can help with tension, posture, energy and flexibility for the day.

Try sitting upright, on the bed or floor, back straight with your legs out in front of you, toes pointing towards the ceiling and arms relaxed down by your sides. **Slowly** begin tilting your head forward, bringing your chin down towards your chest, so you feel a gentle stretch right down your neck and back. Breathe slowly and deeply, feeling the weight of your head helping to stretch those neck and back muscles each time you exhale. When you are ready, as you breathe in, slowly and gently begin raising your head back up to the starting position looking forward.

From there, raise your arms out in front of you, keep your back straight and lean in as far as you can towards your toes to *really* feel the stretch down the back of your legs. Hold for 30 seconds, only focusing on deep, calm breaths in and out.

Next, try the same body position, with legs out in front of you, but reach up as high as you can towards the ceiling, bringing the palms of your hands together and push right into the stretch, remembering to breathe. You will feel the stretch in your arms, shoulders, and down the sides of your back.

While you are in that position, try a little chest and bust boosting exercise. With the palms of your hands still together, bring them down to bust level and push the palms of your hands into each other as hard as you can, holding for 2/3 seconds for each squeeze. Try at least ten reps of these daily for a perk up, it takes less than half a minute!

A FEW MINUTES A DAY IS ALL YOU NEED

Do these stretches and breathing exercises for just a few minutes every morning you will feel the positive effect afterwards! Remember, every movement counts and stretching makes movement a lot easier. Apart from waking up your whole body it will help

Size HH

prepare and encourage you to be more active afterwards! Although stretching is particularly good in the morning, any time of day is beneficial.

By starting the day with stretches like these you will find you instantly have more energy, increased flexibility and better circulation which helps with the natural detox process. Stretching lengthens the muscles keeping you nice and supple and able to move more freely. So next time you wake up, give these simple stretches a go.

Of course, if you wanted to gain the most benefits from stretching, it may be worth learning some proper yoga moves. There is loads of information, pictures, videos and fantastic classes out there to show you how to do everything correctly.

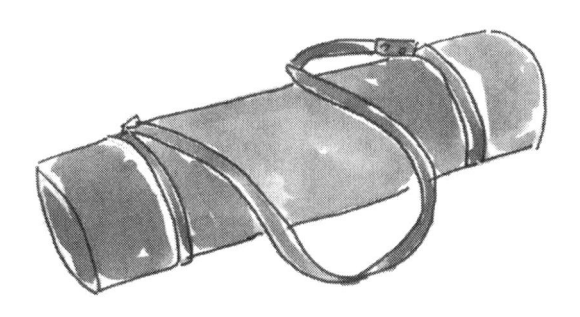

POSTURE

Posture is a sometimes forgotten part of creating a new figure. A good posture can help us appear to lose dress sizes instantly! It makes us feel more confident and influences how others perceive us in a positive way.

How is your posture right now, reading this book?

BREATHE

How we look and feel in our clothes (and out of them) can be affected by posture. If we spend long periods of time sitting down, chances are our posture is suffering for it. Many people experience frequent back pain and other problems due to years of holding bad posture. Not only that, but sitting hunched over regularly can also mean we are only taking shallow breaths for long periods of time which is not great news for our health or wellbeing. Deep breaths cost nothing, and you can do them absolutely anywhere! Anyone can learn better posture, at any age.

Size HH

For instance, sitting for long periods at a desk with the wrong posture can limit your breath and movement as the muscles tighten to hold you in that position. Breathing and posture go hand in hand. So, next time you think about it, take a deep breath, and check you are sitting or standing up straight, with your shoulders back and stomach in.

Correcting your posture is about strengthening and training the right muscles so they begin to do it automatically. Just by practicing to hold the stomach in as often as you can, you will eventually see it becoming flatter and flatter as the muscles become stronger. Hold your stomach in now for as long as you can (remember to breathe).

From now on, every time you think of your 'carrot' motivation, remember to check your posture. Learning good posture is an amazing tool you can use to instantly make you feel and look better. Remember habits become ingrained more quickly and more deeply when you do it with emotion, so revel in the positive effects it has for your body. Feel great about it and practice it several times daily to create a strong habit.

TONING

I have never enjoyed the gym. I personally don't find it the most inspiring way to work out, but I appreciate everyone is different, and some really benefit from it. Plus, after having two children close together in age, I can certainly think of better ways to spend my precious time at the moment. However, I do like to stay fit and energetic, so I had to come up with ways of doing this from home with two toddlers running around.

Toning means more than just tightening the muscles; it means strengthening them too which is excellent for posture. Contrary to popular belief, toning and strengthening isn't just for body builders and doesn't have to be done at the gym.

HOW TO FIT MORE TONING EXERCISES IN TO YOUR CURRENT LIFESTYLE

If you are eating/drinking right, you don't actually have to go too far out of your way to work out. Let's take a look at some ways you can incorporate more health-boosting exercise into your lifestyle right now.

STANDING

As we mentioned before, just the simple act of standing requires the glutes (butt) and thigh muscles to work, so take waiting in a queue, or having to stand on the bus/tube/train as an opportunity to tone! Just tense the glutes and hold for as long as possible, relax and repeat. If you find yourself standing again that day you could mix it up with some short sharp clench and releases, or working on one side at a time. While you are there make sure you are standing up straight, avoiding shallow breathing.

BRUSHING YOUR TEETH

This can provide a double quick workout, simply having your arm in the air while brushing for a few minutes will perk up those arm muscle **if you keep your elbow as high as you can**. If your knees will allow, you could also hold a squat, or hold on to the sink with one hand and try some back leg lifts!

SUPERMARKET

Find a spot in the car park further away from the store than usual and if you have the time, walk every aisle – those extra steps do really add up! Step trackers are a good way to check this. You will be surprised at how quickly a few extra steps add up over the weeks. These are great for challenging your friends and family on how many steps you can do too.

ON YOUR MOBILE

If you enjoy browsing the web/texting whilst lying in bed, or on the sofa for instance, hold the phone away from your body for as long as you can (without dropping the phone on your face!) The more you resist gravity the more you'll tone the muscles and feel the burn as it works.

DRIVING

If you spend a lot of time in the car take this as an opportunity to create a new healthy habit! The whole time you are in the car you can be sitting up right with your back straight, activating your waist, back and stomach muscles (creating a good posture). If you hit some traffic, pass the time with some butt clenches, even challenging yourself to how many you can do before traffic moves again! Hit a red light? Squeeze those glutes as tight as you can until it turns amber! Obviously it defeats the object if you do this while nibbling a packet of something naughty you picked up at the petrol station! Moving swiftly on…

BLOW-DRYING YOUR HAIR

Standing up, (or holding a low squat if you're feeling energetic) rather than sitting down while you blow-dry your hair will really help tighten those thigh and bum muscles. Plus, holding the weight of the hairdryer for a good 10/20 minutes above your head is an arm workout in itself. Just remember to switch arms half way through to keep it even. If you have the time, use the cooler setting for a few extra minutes toning and less damage on the hair.

WALKING IN THE COLD

When it's chilly, our bodies have to work harder to keep its temperature up, burning a few more calories than usual. Plus we tend to tense our muscles more when we are cold so it's a double workout, without even realising!

TAKING A HOT BATH

Sure it's not the same as going for a jog, but the heat, just like the cold, challenges the body to keep its temperature down. It also relieves tension, relaxes the muscles and gives us time to mentally unwind. Just don't go too hot with the water! If you have a minute, tackle the bingo wings with a very simple, one minute arm tone! Sit with good posture, or stand if in the shower and hold a shampoo or shower gel bottle out in front of you, to the side, or behind you (the fuller the better), using it as a weight and hold for as long as you can (at least count to 20) before switching arms. Remember to breathe and keep your back straight, stomach in!

PREPARING FOOD

Mixing, chopping, standing up, lifting saucepans etc. It's all movement, it all counts! Waiting for the microwave to stop? Stand on one leg for as long as you can, then switch. **Never wait for anything again!** These are your little opportunities to make yourself feel good!

Size HH

WATCHING TV

If you like to lay down to watch your favourite programs, challenge yourself (or your friends/family) and do some leg raises at the same time! Simply lay on your back or your side and lift one leg up slowly in front of you as high as you can, then back down as *slowly* as you can, remembering to breathe. Try 5/10 on each leg to start with and build yourself up! Leg raises are great for people with knee conditions or injuries (Of course, always consult your doctor before trying new exercises with any type of body condition or injury.)

CARRYING SHOPPING

Carrying shopping bags can be a great workout. Just remember your back and keep the weight balanced on each side to prevent strain. Tensing your stomach muscles is a good way to bring your back in to line when carrying things. Always bend at the knees when lifting to take the strain off your back.

LAUNDRY

Just the act of carrying heaps of washing in and out, especially when damp, is toning muscles! So remember if you feel exasperated with all the washing, it's helping you out towards your daily exercise too! When bending over to take out the damp washing from the basket to hang up for drying, make sure to take the weight into the hips and legs rather than the back, by bending at the knees (or hips if you have bad knees, with back straight). Stretching up to the washing line with damp clothes is a nice little workout for the arms too! Then, of course, there is the ironing (do it standing up) and putting it all away again too, so you can see this laundry business is starting to look pretty good for your body after all! If you hand wash anything, this is an even better arm, shoulder and back workout!

HOUSEWORK

Mopping, dusting, hoovering, polishing, you name it, it all counts as movement! Cleaning something at a low height? Be sure to either bend from the hips, keeping your back straight (like a door hinge) to work the glutes, or at the knees, like a squat if you can.

UNLOADING/LOADING THE DISHWASHER

Yes, you can make even the most mundane tasks into a chance to release some feel good chemicals and make yourself feel chirpy. Just make sure to take any weight in your legs rather than your back. For women, especially those of us with larger bust, leaning over unloading dishwashers can equal back ache, but by bending your legs at the knees (like squatting), or hips and keeping your back straight, you will save yourself the pain and have a pretty decent workout at the same time.

FOR THOSE OF US THAT DON'T DO DISHWASHERS

Tone up while you do the dishes, or wash the baby's bottles etc, just by doing it standing on one leg for as long as you can, or on tip toes! To really feel the burn, try lifting one leg out behind you as high as you can manage and just hold it there for 10 seconds whilst clenching the buttocks before returning foot to the floor. Repeat as many times as you can handle (or time permits), then switch legs. You can rest your forearms on the sink for balance if needed and still have your hands free.

DANCING/MUSIC

Dancing makes everyone feel great, if there is an opportunity, do it! Stick on your favourite music as you do the housework and boogie your way through it, or join a dance class you have always wanted to try. Even just putting some headphones in and going for a walk can be surprisingly uplifting. Music is definitely a gift worth using if it makes you feel good. Remember, <u>positive feelings bring motivation and energy</u>!

WORK

Sat at your desk for long periods of time? Find a way of creating a regular good posture habit (even if it's a post it note stuck to your computer screen with the letter P on it!) Consciously holding good posture will help tone the right muscles to keep it that way. Do leg, feet and toe movements as you work to keep the blood flowing and try to sit with both feet flat on the ground rather than cross-legged. For tension release, give yourself an upper body and neck a good stretch every hour by twisting slowly from side to side with arms stretched overhead, taking deep breathes as you do so.

BAD KNEES

If you suffer from knee problems, you may find many exercises harder or even impossible. Try sitting in a comfortable chair, preferably one with arm rests you can hold on to. Keep your right foot flat on the floor and stretch your left leg out with your heel resting on the floor and toes pointing towards upwards to ceiling. Begin raising your left leg as high and slowly as you can, then back to the floor as slowly as you can, remembering to breathe. Lightly touch your heel on the floor before slowly raising the leg again for another rep. Try 5/10 to start with, or as many times as you can before switching legs.

BEING ON HOLD

One of my pet hates was being put on hold, now I use it as a few minutes to get something done! Sometimes it's toning my inner thighs… If you want to have a go, start by standing on your left leg, then lift your right foot out in front of you and swing it out over your left leg as high as you can, (gently, minding not to boot the cat at the same time) so that your inner thigh is facing upwards. Hold it there for 2 seconds, then return your right leg back to the start. Repeat 5/10 times then switch legs.

STAIRS

If you have stairs in your house, just going up those a

few times every day (with energy I might add, not just dragging yourself up every step) all factors into your exercise and really helps to build muscle tone, so take any excuse to use them! You probably know what else I am going to say...take the stairs instead of the elevators when you are out and about, because every step counts!

CHANGING BEDS

This dreaded chore can actually be a pretty decent workout without you even realising... All that stretching, plumping, and duvet changing mounts up to a mini toning session for your arms, abs, shoulder, glutes and thigh muscles. Clean bed sheets just got even better!

JUST BEING AT HOME

Need something from another room? Run there, jog there, even skip there if you really want to because it's another opportunity to release some feel good dopamine!

BATHING THE KIDS

Start by kneeling next to the bath, so kids are in full view and arms reach, bottom resting on your heels.

Size HH

Instead of taking all of the weight on your knees, try shifting some of it back onto your shins and feet. Once you have taken some of the weight off your knees, slowly push your whole body weight up using your bottom muscles as far as you can, then back down again slowly and repeat. Honestly, do this at least ten times, really concentrating on firming those butt muscles you will definitely start to feel it working. The kids might think you look funny but nothing wrong with that!

JUST BEFORE YOU SIT DOWN – HOLD IT!

Just as your bottom is an inch away from the chair or sofa and you are about to plonk it down, hold it there for at least 5 seconds. Keep your back straight and remember to breathe. Then sit down. Imagine how quickly this would add up if you did it every time you sat down…

For an extra fat burn, you can try many of these exercises while wearing ankle or arm weights! You can find these at little cost, and they really work. By adding resistance to even the simplest of moves, results will show quicker and give you more of a challenge. Anything that defies gravity is resistance, so even simply holding your arm out in front of you is resisting the pull of gravity. Add some weight to this and the pull will become even stronger.

Combining the right nutrition with stretching, posture and some resistance exercises will give you exceedingly quick results. Results mean more confidence and motivation to keep going! Anyone can do these types of resistance movements, whatever your current physical shape, lifestyle, or beliefs about exercise.

By associating certain tasks with certain exercises like these above, they have become part of my daily routine and habits. This means I can achieve a healthy amount of daily exercise without really thinking about it, or taking much time out of my day for it.

CARDIO

Anyone ready for a heart-racing, sweat-inducing cardio session!? No, me neither.

For many of us, the mere thought of this is off-putting! Though it doesn't have to be as unpleasant, or hard as you may imagine…

Size HH

Exercise releases mood lifting endorphins throughout our body and the more we do, the better we will feel all round. Guaranteed.

Short bursts of cardio (even as little as 40 seconds) every day can really make a positive difference to health, mental wellbeing and fitness levels, allowing you to build yourself up. So if you think you don't have time for long work outs, know that cardio doesn't necessarily have to be long!

Even jogging/running on the spot for 30 seconds a few times per day (even while you wait for the kettle to boil) will help immensely, especially if you have been off exercise for some time.

Brisk walking is an excellent form of cardio and works just as well as running for health benefits, so if you are not into running, don't stress, just start with walking and build yourself up to a fast paced walk. If you took every opportunity to do this, your heart, thigh and bottom muscles would absolutely love you for it! Grab the kids, dog, hubby, friend, your headphones, or just your peace of mind and some water, and find somewhere you would really enjoy a good 10/15 minute brisk walk. If you make your walk as enjoyable as possible, your brain can log some positive emotion with what you are doing and help you turn it into a regular habit you enjoy.

When weather permits, take an hour for a game of tennis, football, frisbee, netball, or volleyball with the kids, family, or friends. We are never too mature for some old-school fun! Many of us forget how invigorating and beneficial fresh air and laughter can be.

Find what works best for you, with cardio especially as it is the one form of exercise many of us try to avoid, but essential for healthy hearts and a superb natural wellbeing boost within minutes. Make it something fun that you enjoy for some **fast** feel good energy. Even running around at home, playing with the kids or dog is better than nothing. If you can really feel your heart beating afterwards, that's a little burst of cardio for you!

Maybe group workouts would bring you more motivation for exercise?

There are so many fab fitness groups to choose from now including; various types of yoga, Pilates, Zumba, aerobics, and spinning classes to name a few.

Size HH

These are not only good for staying motivated with your friends, but also a chance to pick up professional tips you can keep with you for life.

CONCLUSION TO EXERCISE

If you are eating and drinking right, exercise doesn't have to take up much of your life (unless your career is your body like model or body builder etc) and it will become easier and easier if you do it every day. Becoming aware of what exercise you currently do and adding to that where you can, is an easy way to start becoming healthier and happier starting from now.

EXERCISE POINTS TO REMEMBER

- Every step and movement counts! Something is always better than nothing.
- Stretching is the best way to prepare and entice your body into more activity every day. It also helps with toning, circulation and all round better wellbeing!
- From now on, any time you think about the part of your body you dislike, be thankful you have that part of your body and focus on optimum health for it. Instead of disliking it, do a

targeted exercise on it to give yourself a boost, then switch your attention to something you do like about yourself.
- Breathe! Sometimes we naturally hold our breath unconsciously when exercising or take shallow breaths for many hours of the day without realising. Deep breaths cost nothing and you can do them anywhere, at any time and it makes pretty much any task or situation easier.
- Appear more confident and make the most of your figure instantly just by correcting your posture!
- If you are eating the right fuels and less of the rubbish ones, you won't have to do any excessive workouts to lose excess body fat.
- Become more aware of how active you are every day. Step trackers, journals or specialised apps can make easy work of this
- Any movements that use resistance will tone muscles a lot quicker – using any type of weights, even ankle weights, bags of sugar or bottles of water will work. No need for expensive equipment! You can also create

Size HH

resistance with your own body weight or household items by working against gravity.

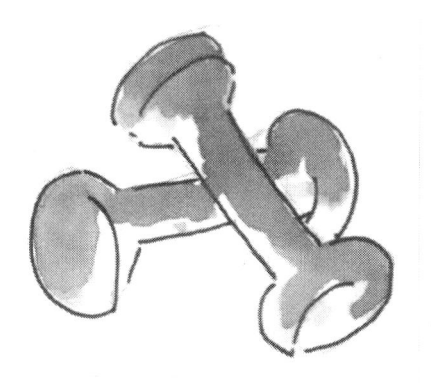

I hope this helps to give you ways of incorporating more mood-boosting, health-provoking exercise into your life, without disrupting your lifestyle!

Eva George

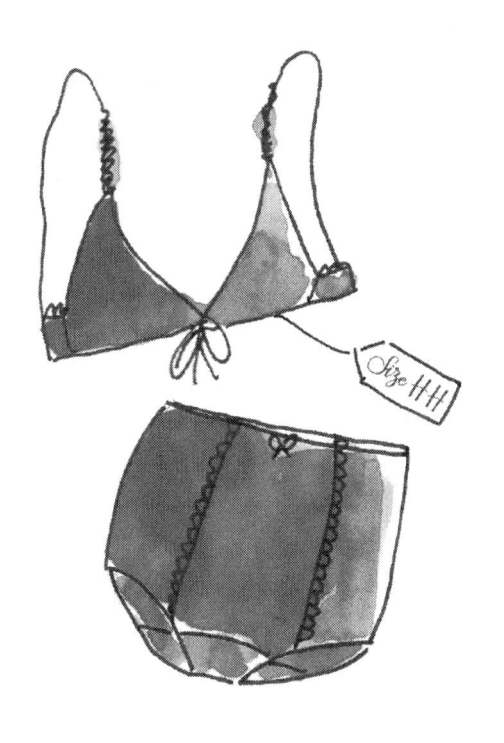

OVERALL POINTS TO REMEMBER

MIND

- Everything starts from your powerful thoughts, use them wisely and make them positive.

LIFESTYLE

- If you want to make parts of your lifestyle healthier, know that you have the ability to make it happen, regardless of your current circumstance.

NUTRITION

- Food and drink is our fuel, but it's also there to be enjoyed. Find your balance and live life happy and diet free!

EXERCISE

- Stretching, deep breathing, and practicing good posture are instant, powerful exercises for your body and wellbeing. Once you have cracked those, you will find yourself looking at your body (and maybe even your day) in a different, more positive way.

Size HH

Well done for investing the time in yourself to read Size HH and thank you for choosing. Once you experience how good it feels to be as healthy as you can be and genuinely content inside your body, life is certainly more enjoyable!

Feel free to update us on your journey to Size Happy & Healthy as you go with our online readers club.

Here is to setting a good example to the younger generations of girls, so they can see from us that it's ok to be different shapes and sizes and by aiming for healthy rather than skinny, their weight won't be an issue, and their unique shape will blossom perfectly. Just like yours can. It is never too late to make healthier choices, become more active, or lose unhealthy body fat that has been holding you back. Now go make a new healthier habit today and please, if you need support or motivation, keep me close so you can refresh with the points to remember pages and feel free to join our ever growing community online.

Eva George

Size HH

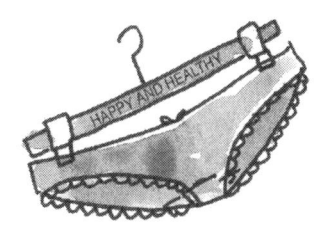

ACKNOWLEDGEMENTS

I would like to start by thanking all the past and present mother figures in my life, including my birth mother of course, for all support, patience, guidance, knowledge, wisdom, inspiration, strength, and love throughout the years that has helped make all this possible in some way or another. Thank you Val

George, Jacqueline Morgan, Tracey Bateman, Sarah George and Jannette Brookman.

Without doubt, one of my biggest thankyous goes to one of my oldest and dearest friends, Carlie Bateman. A fountain of moral support, honest feedback, love and laughter. Late nights of helping me with research and design ideas. This book wouldn't be what it is without this girl.

I would like to thank Mercedez Lopez Charro for being a huge support throughout this process and going way beyond her title of Illustrator, becoming a great friend also. The passion and commitment Mercedes has put into this project is astounding and she has brought the entire thing to life. I can't thank Mercedes enough for her skills and time spent on the project.

Jacqui Malpass has been more than an editor on this project, providing me with a listening ear and professional guidance when I have needed it most. Jacqui has helped me take my message and produce it in the best way I could, bringing out the best in this project, so a big thank you for that Jacqui.

Size HH

Natalie Guyan was originally going to be a short case study but after getting to know her more, I realised just how inspirational she is. Natalie has now become a big part of the Size HH projects and I would like to thank her for all her hard work, strength, guidance and support.

Sarah Arrow deserves a big thank you for creating the Size HH website and putting up with me not having the time to be techy! This women is a complete superstar and has provided top class support in more ways than one.

Caroline Ferguson has been an absolute godsend for this project. Caroline not only provided us with extremely helpful and useable tips and advice, she also helped be back stages with other elements of the book itself. Many thanks and appreciation to Caroline for all her hard work on Size HH.

Thanks to Alison Francis (Sleep Guru) for providing us with great information and tips to use in the book, no questions asked just a giving nature and wonderful woman, thanks Anandi.

Jane Travis, I would like to thank for her contributions to the book, her skills, honesty and no nonsense approach to life.

A big thank you to Georgina Shaw, a former boss of mine who has helped me get the Size HH message out to the world. More than PR, a good friend also and so encouraging every step of the way. Georgina took a big weight off my shoulders without battering an eyelid and I appreciate that immensely!

Ali Meehan, thanks to you and your extensive network of amazing women for your support with the launch!

Tricia Willder, my auntie, I thank for providing moral support, strength and inspiration even from afar.

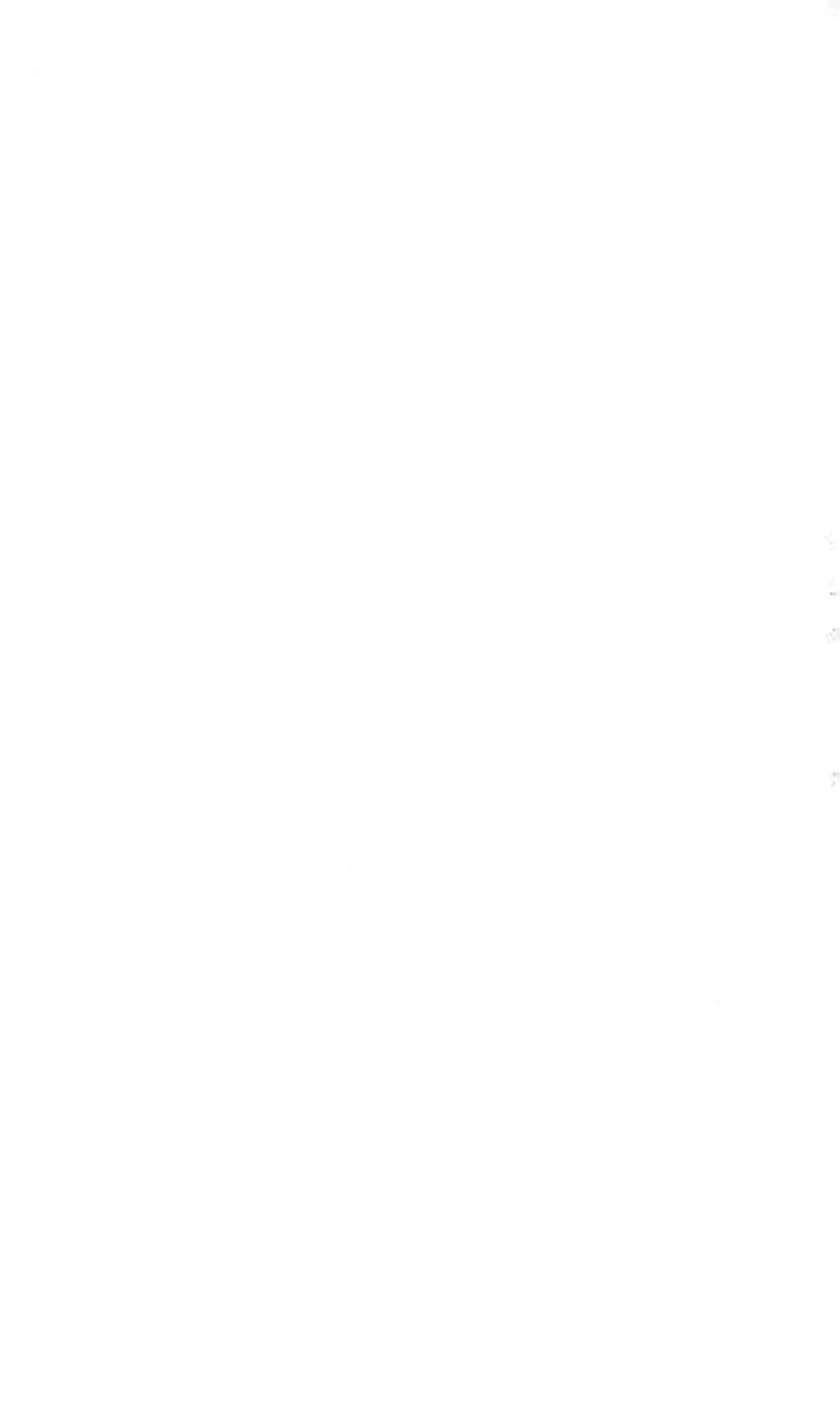

Made in the USA
Charleston, SC
27 March 2016